PSYCHOLOGY OF EMOTIONS, MOTIVATIONS AND ACTIONS

# THE END OF SUICIDOLOGY

## CAN WE EVER UNDERSTAND SUICIDE?

# PSYCHOLOGY OF EMOTIONS, MOTIVATIONS AND ACTIONS

Additional books and e-books in this series can be found on Nova's website under the Series tab.

PSYCHOLOGY OF EMOTIONS, MOTIVATIONS AND ACTIONS

# THE END OF SUICIDOLOGY

## CAN WE EVER UNDERSTAND SUICIDE?

DAVID LESTER

nova science publishers
New York

**Library of Congress Cataloging-in-Publication Data**

ISBN: 978-1-53615-310-1

*Published by Nova Science Publishers, Inc. † New York*

# CONTENTS

# PREFACE

Periodically, researchers express concern about the research conducted on suicide. Back in 1966, Merton Kahne criticized the quality of the research, but more recently, some scholars have declared that we have reached our limits in understanding and predicting suicide. Dan Reidenberg recently wrote an editorial entitled "Healthy debate, frustration, or a field in chaos?" in which he discussed the failure in the United States to reduce the suicide rate (which in recent years has been rising). Cas Soper has argued that there is no empirical reason to believe that predictors of suicide exist, there is no theoretical foundation for believing that risk factors exist, and there is evidence that suicide may be predictably unpredictable!

David Lester reviews and discusses these views in *The End of Suicidology: Can We Ever Understand Suicide?* He reviews some recent efforts to stimulate the field of suicidology, and finds these attempts lacking. In the major section of the book, Lester presents some recent provocative ideas on suicide that have not hitherto received much attention, such as Brian Mishara's two component model of suicide with life and suicide tendencies, and David Lester and Steven Stack's proposal that suicide may be viewed as a drama staged by the prospective suicide. Might these provocative ideas and others stimulate the field?

In: The End of Suicidology
Editor: David Lester
ISBN: 978-1-53615-310-1


*Chapter 1*

# THE END OF SUICIDOLOGY[1]

***David Lester, PhD***
Stockton University, Galloway, New Jersey, US

The end of the 20th Century produced an interesting trend in the scholarly field – a sense that everything was coming to an end. Francis Fukuyama (1992) declared that history had come to an end and that little of importance would happen in the future. David Lindley (1994) followed with a declaration that physics had discovered all that was to be discovered, and John Horgan (1997a) declared that science, in general, had solved all of the puzzles.

Horgan argued that pure science had entered its twilight, that is, there are no more profound revelations that will occur. He noted that science as a whole was not ending, but that *path-breaking* science was ending. Horgan (1997b) also suggested that even applied science might be endling. After all, he noted, where are the nuclear fusion reactors that were predicted in the 1950s? Has the war on cancer declared by President Richard Nixon in 1972 been won yet?

[1] Adapted from Lester (2000a, 2000b).

I taught courses on Theories of Personality and Theories of Psychotherapy, and the same seems to be true in those fields too. The last major theory of personality was from George Kelly and published in 1955., and the last major systems of psychotherapy stemmed from Albert Ellis and Fritz Perls in the 1960s and Arthur Janov in the 1970s. Since then, a degree in marketing would be more appropriate than a degree in psychology, for the so-called "new theories" proposed have been little more than a re-packaging of the older theories, combined in a new mix and with new terms for old concepts.

What of suicidology? Every 10 years for the 30 years I reviewed the suicidology research and theories as completely and extensively as I could (Lester, 1972, 1983, 1992, 2000), covering the years 1897-1997. There was an obvious conclusion from the 4th review in 1997. Nothing of importance had been published in the 1990s. Indeed, for each decade, I selected the major contributions to the field of suicidology, such as Edwin Shneidman in the 1960s, Aaron Beck and David Phillips in the 1970s. They introduced new topics and research foci for suicidology and produced a large body of work on those topics. There was no one, in my opinion, worthy to be chosen for the 1990s, and my perusal of suicide research and theory since then finds no major contributor to the field in the last 20 years.

The topics for research in suicidology these days are those that had been identified earlier. Indeed, it is depressing to see the same kinds of research being conducted as has been published many times before. A large sample of subjects is administered scales for depression, hopelessness, self-esteem, life stress and other variables in order to predict suicidal behavior using a multiple regression model. Or a sample of suicidal subjects is examined for psychiatric characteristics. (How many more times must we read that comorbidity is a risk factor for suicide?) Or a set of social indicators is (again) entered into a multiple regression analysis to predict suicide rates over time in nations or over regions. Or a few brains are examined for a dozen or so biochemicals in up to 30 or so brain regions. In this latter example, not only are the results inconsistent, but it is often apparent that the published paper on suicide is a side issue since the initial goal of the research was to study depression or schizophrenia, but the investigators saw that they could produce an additional paper or two by studying the suicides in the sample.

In addition,some topics in suicidology have been *removed* for our purview, topics such as sex differences in suicidal behavior or the variation of suicide over the menstrual cycle. It is not that we actually tested and confirmed theories of these phenomena. It seems rather that we simply lost interest. For example, with regard to sex differences in suicidal behavior, despite the many papers and books on the topic, there have been almost no empirical tests of theories of the sex difference. Rather, we read mere *discussions* of the topic. This was especially true of the female suicide rate in China which was higher than the male suicide rate for many years. Dozens of papers appeared that noted this difference (almost all using the same WHO data), speculating on the causes of this difference. Yet few, if any, papers attempted to test a theory for this difference.

In the 1990s (and still today), a number of suicidologists argued that we needed a meaningful and generally agreed-upon terminology for suicidology, and several papers have appeared on this topic (e.g., O'Carroll, et al., 1996). In my opinion, there is no urgent need for a new terminology. Rather, what we need are good theories, especially good competing and incompatible theories, and methodologically sound empirical tests of these competing theories.

## Research on Individuals

Research on individuals has been limited by the psychiatric diagnostic system. First, this diagnostic system is not etiological, that is, based on causes. The medical system, in general (but not always), assesses symptoms and then tries to locate the underlying cause. Is the headache and fever a result of influenza, malaria, diverticulitis, etc.? There is no "illness" labelled headache/fever. In contrast, the psychiatric diagnostic system is based on clusters of symptoms and not on causes.[2] This lack of psychiatric disorders with a clear etiology makes the psychiatric diagnostic system unscientific and of little use for understanding suicide.

In addition, research is often methodologically unsound because the researchers fail to control for diagnosis. For example, studies of childhood sexual abuse do find an association with later suicidal behavior. But, is this link direct or is it mediated by psychiatric disturbance? Childhood sexual abuse results in an increase in all kinds of disorders, such as substance abuse, eating disorders and depression. Perhaps it is these conditions that increase the risk of suicidal behavior?

Apart from research on psychiatric patients, a great deal of psychological research on suicidal behavior focuses on suicidal ideation (and occasionally suicide attempts) in university students. This is because many researchers are academics and, therefore, have easy access to students and, in addition, are under pressure to publish (or perish). Not only does this result in multiple regressions of clusters of variables predicting suicidal ideation (as criticized above), but the research may have little implication for completed suicide.[3] Of course, the role of psychological variables is impossible to explore in those who are dead, but psychological autopsy studies of those who have died by suicide constitute more meaningful studies of the causes of suicide than studies of students with suicidal ideation.

As far as theorizing about suicide, two comments are relevant. First, most of the research into suicide ignores the major theories of human behavior, commonly known as theories of personality[4] and systems of psychotherapy. These fundamental theories of human behavior need to be brought into the study of suicide. Second, almost all research that seeks to test psychological theories of suicide typically test only one theory. It is rare for research to compare and contrast two theories, ideally two theories that are incompatible with each other.

---

[2] Of course, there are those medical illnesses prefaced by the term "idiopathic" which means that the physician does not know the cause, as well as diseases such as colitis, which merely mean some problem in the colon.

[3] I, too, have been guilty of this.

[4] *Theories of the mind* would be a more appropriate term than *theories of personality*.

## Sociological Research

Consider Durkheim's (1897) theory. In Durkheim's theory, there are four types of suicide based on two dimensions: social integration and social regulation. Two dimensions provide a zonal analysis with types such as high social integration plus low social regulation, etc. These four types do *not* match Durkheim's four types: egoistic suicide resulting from low social integration, altruistic suicide resulting from high social integration, anomic suicide resulting from low social regulation, and fatalistic suicide resulting from high social regulation. Durkheim never considered these two dimensions of social integration and social regulation at the same time.

Rootman (1973) noted this and reported a preliminary study, rating a sample of primitive societies for three levels of each dimensions (low, moderate and high) and looking at estimated suicide rates for the societies in each of the nine cells of the 3-by-3 array. Lester1989) reported a similar analysis using developed nations. These studies have been ignored. Instead, sociologists examine simple correlations of variables such as divorce rates and female labor force participation with suicide rates. They never even investigate whether divorce rates or female labor force participation are empirically associated with Durkheim's concepts of social integration and social regulation. Are divorced people less socially integrated or socially regulated than married people? I have never seen a study on this. Furthermore, sociologists study the *total suicide rate*, whereas Durkheim's theory requires that the research study the anomic, egoistic, altruistic and fatalistic suicide rates separately.

A further problem with Durkheim's theory is that it has acquired the status of a "religion" and anyone who changes it is labelled as a heretic. This process impedes scientific progress. One reviewer rejected an article of mine on Durkheim because I also included homicide as a dependent variable, and Durkheim did not do this. Another reviewer rejected an article I had submitted because it was on primitive societies and, again, Durkheim did not study primitive societies.

## JOINER'S THEORY OF SUICIDE

A word is appropriate here about Thomas Joiner's Interpersonal Theory of Suicide (ITS) which, in the 2010s, has become the basis for much research in suicidology. Surely this theory an antidote to the criticisms of suicidology raised above? Joiner's theory proposed that two constructs were important in motivating suicide: thwarted belongingness and perceived burdensomeness. In addition, the potential suicide also had to develop an acquired capability for suicide, including such traits as a tolerance for pain and a reduced fear of death.

The ITS (Joiner, 2007) has received a lot of criticism, both in print (e.g., Paniagua, et al. 2010) and informally among suicidologists. The two major criticisms are that it is not new (Durkheim already proposed thwarted belongingness) and that it is dominating the field. Both are unfair. Let us first look at whether it is new.

To be sure, thwarted belongingness is not new. Durkheim's concept of social integration is somewhat similar to thwarted belongingness, but actually Raoul Naroll's concept of *thwarting disorientation* (Lester, 1995) is closer to thwarted belongingness. Anyway, using the ideas of earlier people in the field is not a sin. One of my brilliant professors at Cambridge University, Richard Gregory, whose field was perception, admitted that he spent a great deal of time reading German scholars from the late 1800s and then "re-discovering" their insights in modern times. For example, he "discovered" a wonderful crustacean in the Mediterranean that scanned the environment with one receptor, much as television cameras did.

However, not only was the concept of perceived burdensomeness not a focus of research prior to the ITS, but the concept of the acquired capability for suicide was also barely mentioned in the literature, if at all. As the singer *Meatloaf* has said in a different context, two out of three ain't bad. No one else has developed a new theory or opened a new area of research in recent years. I think that the concept of thwarted belongingness could be modified to make it more useful and relevant, but the focus of the ITS on burdensomeness and the acquired capability is innovative.

One valid criticism of the concept of perceived burdensomeness is that the ITS implies that it is present in *all* suicides in *all* cultures, and this is much too extreme. It may be present in some suicides, but not in all. If it is not involved in all suicides, then the theory is limited, and even modifications to the theory by bringing in other variables cannot fully remedy this. In addition, rather than being a new *theory*, the ITS can be viewed as merely adding *additional risk factors*.

As for the domination of the theory, there are two relevant objections to complaining about this. First, it is clear that most current researchers in suicidology rarely read (and, therefore, cite) research and theory prior to the year 2000. The use of online searching through PsycInfo and PubMed force this since the most recent articles come up first and because the literature on suicide is now immense. No one has the time (or the motivation) to scroll down to earlier years. Furthermore, without anyone thoroughly reviewing the field since my last review in 1997, there is no easy source for finding out what has been written in the past. The current domination of the ITS is, therefore, understandable. People are not finding and reading earlier alternative theories.

Second, if the domination of the ITS is irritating, then come up with an alternative. It is always easier to criticize than to provide an alternative. If those critics of the domination of the ITS could propose an alternative theory, then, of course, they would do so. A new theory would be exciting, but I am not holding my breath in anticipation of it.

## A Devastating Meta-Analysis

I have criticized research, but is there any evidence to back up my criticism. Franklin, et al. (2016) published a meta-analysis of research on risk factors for suicidality that provides evidence for the failure of current suicidology research. At the beginning of their review, Franklin et al defined risk factors.

A *correlate* is a variable that is associated with another variable. For example, if I were to give a scale to measure hopelessness and a question to assess current suicidal ideation to a sample of undergraduate students in my college class, the two scores would most likely be associated. This type of study is called a cross-sectional study. A *risk factor* requires a longitudinal (follow-up) design. I would give the scale to measure hopelessness at the beginning of the semester and measure current suicidal ideation at the end of the semester. If the scores prove to be associated (or correlated), then I can say that hopelessness at time 1 predicts suicidal ideation at time 2. This makes hopelessness a risk factor. A *causal risk factor* requires, in addition, that the variable at time 1 causes the variable at time 2. This is much more difficult to establish because, at the present time, there are no *necessary* or *sufficient* variables (or factors) that are known to cause suicidal behavior.

Franklin, et al. also distinguished between statistically significant findings and clinically significant findings. If a research takes a sample of sufficiently large numbers of individuals, it is possible to find statistically significant associations that are so small that they have little clinical (personal or social) significance.

For their meta-analysis, Franklin, et al. found 365 scholarly papers that were able to identify predictive risk factors for suicidal behaviors. These papers produced 3,923 associations of which 3,428 were risk factors and 495 protective factors. Their results can be summarized as below.

| | | |
|---|---|---|
| Suicidal ideation | 572 effect sizes | odds ratio 1.50 |
| Suicide attempts | 1,281 effect sizes | odds ratio 1.51 |
| Completed suicide | 912 effect sizes | odds ratio 1.50 |

All of these mean effect sizes were statistically significant.

Franklin et al. concluded that prediction was only slightly better than chance, no broad category of potential risk factors (such as demographics and physical illness) proved to be better than others, and the predictive ability of the variables had not improved over the 50 years of research.

Let us look at why the significant odds ratios are not evidence of great success. The odds ratio for completed suicide means that the use of the risk factors would increase the one-year odds of a suicidal death would improve from 13 per 100,000 people to 19 or, for one single individual, from 0.00013 to 0.00019. We might note that, in addition to the problems identified by Franklin et al., it has long been noted that the use of any predictive scale (or scales) for predicting suicide would create far too many false positives (that is, individuals predicted to die by suicide but who did not) to be of use. Let us say that we could predict suicide with 75% accuracy (and that would be an incredibly good predictive instrument). Assume that we have a population of 100,000 people (at colleges or in prisons, for example). With a suicide rate of 20 per 100,000 per year (roughly the suicide rate of men in the United States), we would correctly identify 15 of the suicides and, hence, intervene. However, 24,995 non-suicidal individuals would be identified as potential suicides and would have to be placed on suicide watch. These false positives make the situation unfeasible. If the prediction power rose to 90%, there would be 9,9998 false positives.

## Discussion

I was not the first person to criticize "current" suicidology. Back in 1966 Merton Kahne commented negatively on the suicide research of his era.

> The monotonous regularity with which the same types of data are reported and the same stereotyped conclusions inferred from information organized in a fashion whose methodological error has long been demonstrated is only too rarely broken by original ventures beyond the conventional. Indeed, most of the literature does not even qualify as research in the sense of any deliberate hypothesis testing or careful evaluation of the theoretical alternatives implicit in a specific set of events associated with a suicide or group of suicides. Polemics alternate with appeals to the self-evident nature of assumptions. Abbreviated reports do not even have a focal point of common reference. This apathetic caricature of scientific contribution is the most obvious single fact emerging from a reasonably conscientious review of the medical suicide literature. (p. 182)

I liked this so much that I included this paragraph in my first review of the suicidology literature (Lester, 1972). In addition, at that time, elections for the President of the American Association of Suicidology had only one candidate (Lester, 1970), so I wrote in Merton Kahne for President and, at the annual meeting, his single vote was announced to the consternation of those present.

I am not the only suicidologist concerned about the state of the field. Reidenberg (2018) recently wrote an editorial entitled "Healthy debate, frustration, or a field in chaos?" in which he expressed views that are compatible with mine. Reidenberg described a scenario (which actually occurred) in which a bereaved father whose son died by suicide offered $100 million to prevent suicide. What would we do with that money? One debate over how to spend this money that Reidenberg mentioned was that between focusing on high-risk suicidal individuals versus targeting the population as a whole, a debate that Lester and Yang (2006) discussed many years ago. (Note, the two approaches are not incompatible unless one's resources are limited.) Reidenberg's essay focused on the criterion of the United States (or any country) consistently reducing the incidence of suicide. I prefer a criterion of having good theories of suicidal behavior backed up by sound research, regardless of whether they help us prevent suicide.

Soper (2019) has also criticized the search for risk factors that are believed to produce suicide. Soper is convinced that the search will fail, in the same that chemists failed to find phlogiston in the 17$^{th}$ and 18$^{th}$ centuries, the element that was supposed to be released when a substance is burned. Soper argued that there is no empirical reason to believe that predictors of suicide exist, there is no theoretical foundation for believing that risk factors exist, and there is evidence that suicide may be predictably unpredictable. Soper cited the meta-analysis of Franklin, et al. (2017) discussed above and the meta-analyses of others that came to the conclusion that necessary and sufficient, and empirically useful, risk factors have not been identified.

Soper argued that pain is necessary biologically to help animals avoid dangerous situations. Pain is, therefore, aversive, and animals seek to seize opportunities to avoid pain. Humans have developed an intellect that conceived of suicide as a way of avoiding pain. However, natural selection has resulted in sub-groups of the population with a lower rate of suicide surviving and supplanting sub-groups with a higher rate of suicide. Humans, therefore, now have a low, but non-zero, rate of suicide which is unpredictable (see Chapter 10 below). For Soper, suicide is not a deviant behavior but rather an expected by-product of normal human cognition.

I have always been impressed by the complexity of Henry and Short's (1954) theory of suicide and homicide, regardless of how well it predicts and explains suicidal behavior. It has many assumptions, proposes many hypotheses, and cleverly interweaves psychological and sociological concepts.[5] In contrast, psychological models of suicidal behavior imply (by using multiple regression techniques) that suicidal behavior is simply a result of a weighted sum of various psychological traits and states - a little bit of hopelessness plus a little bit of stress, plus…., etc. No interaction terms, nor tests of theories of the form $(A + B^2)/(\sqrt{C} - \log D)$.

So, is it the end of suicidology? I think so, but I hope not. My goal in this book is first to review the work by three groups of suicidologists who have endeavored to provide a stimulus to new research and theory. Secondly, I will present some innovative ideas proposed by myself and others to show that creative research and theorizing in suicidology is still possible.

Before moving on, however, let me mention a brilliant study which I believe all suicide researchers should know about. It is not on suicide, but on murder. Palmer (1960) wanted to study the childhood and adolescent experiences of murderers. He obtained a sample of murderers and compared their lives with the lives of their brothers, using interviews with the murderers, their brothers and their parents. Palmer found significant differences, and the choice of his comparison group (non-murdering brothers) controlled for many confounding variables. I have been disappointed that this methodology has never been used for a study of suicides. I have never found a study comparing a sample of suicides with their siblings.

---

[5] Murderers would make an excellent comparison group of suicides, but I have found only two studies that compared suicides and murderers.

## References


Durkheim, E. (1897). *Le suicide* [*Suicide*]. Paris, France: Felix Alcan.

Franklin, J. C., Robeiro, J. D., Fox, K. R., Bentley, K. H., Kleinman, E. M. & Nock, M. K. (2016). Risk factors for suicidal thoughts and behavior. *Psychological Bulletin, 143,* 187-232.

Fukuyama, F. (1992). *The end of history and the last man*. New York: Free Press.

Henry, A. F. & Short, J. F. (1954). *Suicide and homicide*. New York: Free Press.

Horgan, J. (1997a). *The end of science*. New York: Broadway Books.

Horgan, J. (1997b). Facing up to the decline of science. *Chronicle of Higher Education, 43*(40), A52.

Joiner, T. E. (2007). *Why people die by suicide*. Cambridge, MA: Harvard University Press.

Kahne, M. (1966). Suicide research. *International Journal of Social Psychiatry*, *12*, 177-196.

Lester, D. (1970). The American Association of Suicidology. *Crisis Intervention*, *2*, 30-31. (available at www.drdavidlester.net).

Lester, D. (1972, 1983, 1992, 2000). *Why people kill themselves*. Springfield, IL: Charles Thomas.

Lester, D. (1989). *Suicide from a sociological perspective*. Springfield, IL: Charles Thomas.

Lester, D. (1995). Thwarting disorientation and suicide. *Cross-Cultural Research*, *29*, 14-26.

Lester, D. (2000a). The end of suicidology. *Crisis*, *21*, 158-159.

Lester, D. (2000b). Decades of suicide research. In T. Joiner & M. D. Rudd (Eds.) *Suicide science*, pp. 9-16. Boston: Kluwer.

Lester, D. & Yang, B. (2006). Should suicide prevention programs target individuals or society as a whole? *Crisis*, *27*, 200-201.

Lindley, D. (1994). *The end of physics*. New York: Basic Books.

O'Carroll, P. W., Berman, A. L., Maris, R. W., Mosicki, E., Tanney, B. L. & Silverman, M. (1996). Beyond the Tower of Babel. *Suicide & Life-Threatening Behavior*, *26*, 237-252.

Palmer, S. (1960). *A study of murder*. New York: Thomas Crowell.

Paniagua, F. A., Black, S. A., Gallaway, M. S. & Coombs, M. A. (2010). *The Interpersonal-Psychological Theory of attempted and completed suicide.* Bloomington, IN: Authorhouse.

Reidenberg, D. (2018). Healthy debate, frustration, or a field in chaos? *Crisis*, *39*, 77-81.

Rootman, I. (1973). A cross-cultural note on Durkheim's theory of suicide. *Life-Threatening Behavior*, *3*, 83-94.

Soper, C. A. (2019). Beyond the search for *suigiston*: How evolution offers oxygen for suicidology. In V. Ziegler-Hill & T. K. Shackelford (Eds.) *Evolutionary perspectives on death*. New York: Springer.

# PROPOSED NEW APPROACHES

In: The End of Suicidology
Editor: David Lester ISBN: 978-1-53615-310-1


*Chapter 2*

# KRAL AND WHITE: CRITICAL SUICIDOLOGY

***David Lester, PhD***
Stockton University, Galloway, New Jersey, US

A recent movement, called *critical suicidology* (criticalsuicidology.net) proposes a new approach to understanding suicide (White, et al., 2016). As stated on the website (criticalsuicidology.net):

> Critical Suicidology presents an approach to understanding, theorising and intervening in suicide from alternative perspectives that seek new ways to thinking about suicide from a critical perspective to help address suicide where traditional approaches have failed.

The website lists several critical papers. Broz (2015) stressed the need to have the humanities disciplines and other disciplines contribute to suicidology. He favored qualitative methodologies, and he hoped for more anthropological studies of suicide in the future. But Broz also questioned the focus of the field on two goals: increasing academic knowledge and having a social impact. He suggested that the desire to have a social impact may impede the acquisition of knowledge. I agree with this. One way in which this is manifest in suicidology is the change over the years in the reaction of the suicide organizations and conferences to assisted suicide. Thirty years ago, the American Association of Suicidology invited speakers such as Thomas Szasz and Derek Humphry to debate whether suicide should indeed be prevented and whether do-it-yourself guides to suicide should be encouraged. Later, a move to change the name of the organization to the American Association for Suicide Prevention was fortunately withdrawn. Today, the desire to have a social impact, that is, to *prevent suicide*, has narrowed the debate in the organizations and conferences.

Cover (2016) argued that individuals from the dominant culture cannot understand suicide among the marginalized in the society, including indigenous peoples, refugees, and LGBQT individuals. He also stressed the importance of cultural approaches.

> Cultural…..approaches to understanding both marginality and suicidality permit us to expand on the notion of social and environmental causality by sponsoring a critique of belonging through concepts of different forms of relationality and how they come to bear on the conditions for liveability. (p. 105)

Cover (2013), in his analysis of suicide in "queer" youth, focused on oppression from within the LGBQT community, where norms apparently exist for approved roles in the LGBTQ community. One of the critical questions, I will argue in this book, for the "new approaches" to suicidology is whether they generate new theories. Oppression, and its concomitants, is not a new concept. It is present in Durkheim's (1897) construct of fatalistic suicide, and I have explored the role of oppression in greater depth than in Durkheim's footnote (Lester, 2014a).

Hjelmeland (2010) argued forcefully for cultural and qualitative studies in suicidology. Kral (1998) made a similar argument, noting that individuals typically internalize cultural norms and values and that these influence the decision to die by suicide. Kral also noted that, although it is popular to say that a multidimensional perspective is important in understanding suicide, it is rare for a truely multidimensional model to appear. We might note that it is hard to envision what a multidimensional model might look like. It would not be easy to integrate biological, psychiatric, psychological, social and cultural variables into one model other than putting each set of variables into individual boxes with arrows from each box pointing toward "suicidal behavior," which would amount to little more than saying that suicide is a multidimensional phenomenon.

White (2015, p. 2) stated that it was unimaginable that modern suicidology (and the major suicidology journals) would explore "subjugated meanings of suicide, including for example, suicide as sin, weapon, freedom, philosophical contemplation, or aesthetic experience." She also noted that she had a proposed conference presentation rejected for being political. Lester (1990) described how suicide can be a political act and later discussed suicide as a response to oppression (Lester, 2014a). Lester (2010, 2011) has written on female suicide bombers who clearly use suicide as a weapon. Lester and Stack (2015) wrote a book on suicide as a dramatic performance, which, in part, dealt with the esthetic aspects of suicide. Thus, contrary to White's statement, these ways of viewing suicide are far from "subjugated."

White continued by arguing that suicide is always seen from a psychiatric (mental illness) perspective and is viewed as an act that must be prevented. Of course, many suicidologists fit into this group, but many do not. In addition to people such as Derek Humphry (1991) and Thomas Szasz (1986) who have argued against suicide prevention and in favor of assisted suicide, Lester (2003), in his book *Fixin' to Die*, subtitled it, "A compassionate guide to committing suicide or staying alive," and has talked of suicide as a rational act. Lester (2014c) addressed the rationality of suicide in his book *Rational suicide: Is it possible?*

White also cites a book by Jaworski (2014) entitled *The Gender of Suicide*, which White characterizes as showing how suicidology is a "highly gendered project that depends on dominant cultural (i.e., "masculinist") discourses for its meaning, authority and intelligibility (pp. 203). Such a statement ignores the work of Canetto and Lester (1995) and, even earlier Lester (1989, 1997).

## SOME EXAMPLES

### White and Kral (2014)

White and Kral (2014) set out to provide a new perspective on suicide in youths. They first noted that the major approach to youth suicide (as is the case for suicide in all groups) is individualistic. Personality traits, in particular psychiatric symptoms and disorders, dominate explanations of why people die by suicide, while the impact of social relationship and cultural factors is ignored. To a large extent this true. In his first review of research on suicide from 1897 to 1969 (*Why People Kill Themselves*), Lester (1972) found that there were several studies of relational factors in suicide, particularly in dissertations. For example, Hattem (1964) studied individuals who had attempted or threatened suicide *and* their spouses and explored the role of discordant relationships in suicidal behavior. Peck (1965) examined the role of double-bind communications in the relationships of those who made suicidal gestures. Interestingly, neither of these dissertations were published in scholarly journals. Of course, not all this research remained unpublished. For example, Jacobs's dissertation in 1967 on the progressive disintegration in the social lives of adolescents who attempted suicide appeared as a book (Jacobs, 1971). However, in the later editions of *Why People Kill Themselves,* which reviewed suicide research over the previous ten years, there were fewer and fewer studies of this type after the 1960s. Cynically, we could point to the pressures put on academic researchers to publish in large quantities in the leading scholarly journals. The intense work involved in studying both partners in a marriage or both the child and the parents slows down the quantity of publications and results in less prestigious publications.

White and Kral focused on three cases of suicide, including that of Amanda Todd, who died by suicide after posting on the Internet a video in which she displayed a series of flash cards containing her message (see Lester, McSwain & Gunn, 2013). Amanda had been sexually exploited and, subsequently, harassed by other on social media. White and Kral noted, therefore, the importance of social relationships in her suicide and they cast her use of social media to display her distress as "culturally resonant means of expressing distress" (p. 129).

The question to ask here is whether White and Kral have presented a new theory of adolescent suicide. I think not. The variables discussed (sexual abuse and cyberbullying, or as Amanda's mother prefers cyber-harassment) have been studied by others. What is interesting to note is that White and Kral did not study, nor speculate upon, the role played by Amanda's relationships with her mother, her other family members, and her friends and acquaintances. Amanda's death makes it impossible to study these relationships directly, but cases of adolescents attempting suicide and surviving would provide an opportunity. In their article, White and Kral present a polemic, but they do not present research or a new theory.

## White (2012)

White (2012) stated that she will present a constructionist perspective on suicide, "constituted through language and other relational practices" (p. 42). It is interesting to note that, as regards language, others (but not the critical suicidologists) have devoted much attention to the language used in suicidology. The use of the word *suicide* as a verb (to suicide) is no longer acceptable; nor is *commit suicide*, which tends to cast suicide as a crime (analogous to *committing murder*). There has been debate over the term *survivors of suicide*, which refers to those who have lost a loved one to suicide and not to those who have attempted suicide but survived the attempt. There was also a move to use the word *parasuicide* to label non-lethal suicide attempts (*gestures*). But this is not what White is referring to. She does quote Marsh (2010) who admits that there are, after all, dead bodies, but language does not appear to come into White's thesis.

For theory, White proposed that suicide should be viewed as a *wild problem* which she defines as complex, contextually embedded, uncertain and impossible to predict. The terms complex, uncertain and impossible to predict do not describe a theory. They describe a non-theory. Contextually embedded (although critical suicidologists rare, if ever, define what they mean by *context*), is not a new idea. Context is found in Durkheim's (1897) four-fold classification of suicide, and Richman's (1986) family therapy approach, to name just a couple of theoretical approaches. White also argued that suicide is historically contingent, a truism. Of course, suicide is historically contingent in many ways, from the means chosen for suicide, the views of the society about suicide (as a sin, as the result of a psychiatric disorder, etc.), the motives for suicide, and even the way in which a suicide note is written (on paper versus online using YouTube for suicide notes and live video streaming of the actual suicidal act).

## CONCLUSION

Kouri (2015) noted a feeling of exclusion in some of those working in suicidology in many ways:

> At the level of professional organizations, state science projects a unified field by silencing or recuperating aberrant researchers, dissonant findings, and itinerant practitioners. (p. 67)

He cited scholars who are members of the critical suicidology group who had papers rejected by conferences and from journals. All of us, critical suicidologists or not, radical or not, have had papers rejected by journal editors and submissions rejected by conference chairs. The list of papers and chapters on the critical suicidology website shows that publication is possible, and, of course, it is always possible to establish a new journal for one's perspective. *Suicidology Online* is not critical or radical, but was easily set up, open access, online.

Kouri also illustrates a strong tendency of those who feel excluded to couch their arguments and views in impenetrable jargon. Kouri, of course, is not alone in this criticism, but he does illustrate it himself.

> These autopoetic processes produce experiences of being a self through the folding and unfolding of political, economic, discursive, and other forces. Importantly, the body always subjectifies through its

> relationship to other bodies and social formations and hence through a contingent and perpetually changing exteriority. (Kouri, 2015, p. 69)

Does this have any real meaning?

It is easy to argue that a particular perspective or approach to suicidology has been neglected, or even ignored, but it far from easy to propose an *alternative theory*. Have the critical suicidologists come up with a new model, or even a new variable, to stimulate research into suicide? I would argue that they have not – as yet. As for the role of qualitative research, that type of research can be of interest in understanding suicide in a particular person or a particular culture. But then what? Psychotherapists study individual patients and sometimes publish reports on them. What makes their papers important is when the paper stimulates a hypothesis about suicide.

For example, in my study of Katie's diary (Lester, 2004), I gave the last year of a diary written by a female undergraduate to colleagues and asked them to write about her. Many of the chapters were qualitative. Canetto (2004) picked up the improvement in Katie's mood over the last few months prior to her suicide. A quantitative study by Pennebaker and Stone (2004) confirmed this by counting the words indicating positive and negative emotions. This then raised the question of how common this change in mood over months prior to a suicide might be. Lester (2014b) tested this using several other diaries that he had obtained. Here is a case study leading to a hypothesis and research.

Kral and White (2017, p. 1) have said that critical suicidology "highlights some of the limits of mainstream approaches to embrace more contextualized, poetic, subjective, historical, ecological, social justice oriented, and political perspectives." Marsh (2014) asserted that "Accepting that suicide is as much a social justice issue as a mental health one would require a substantial change in the way we think, but it would open up new possibilities for action," but he gave no indication of what change and what new possibilities.

Here is a challenge to the critical suicidologists. Show me a new theory (or even a new insight) as a result of this approach.

## REFERENCES

Broz, L. (2015). I, too, have a dream … about suicidology. *Social Epistemology Review & Reply Collective*, *4*(7), 27-31.

Canetto, S. S. (2004). Why did you kill yourself, Katie? In D. Lester (Ed.) *Katie's diary*, pp. 41-54. New York: Brunner-Routledge.

Canetto, S. S. & Lester, D. (Eds.) (1995). *Women and suicidal behavior*. New York: Springer.

Cover, R. (2013). Conditions of living. *Journal of LGBT Youth*, *10*, 328-350.

Cover, R. (2016). Suicides of the marginalised: cultural approaches to suicide, relationality and mobility. *Cultural Studies Review*, *22*(2), 90-113.

Durkheim, E. (1897). *Le suicide* [*Suicide*]. Paris, France: Felix Alcan.

Hattem, J. V. (1964). Precipitating role of discordant relationships in suicidal behavior. *Dissertation Abstracts*, *25*, 1336-1336.

Hjelmeland, H. (2010). Cultural research in suicidology: challenges and opportunities. *Suicidology Online*, *1*, 34-52.

Humphrey, D. (1991). *Final exit*. New York: Dell.

Jacobs, J. (1971). *Adolescent suicide*. Oxford, UK: Wiley-Interscience.

Jaworski, K. (2014). *The gender of suicide*. Burlington, VT: Ashgate.

Kouri, S. (2015). Nomad suicidology. *Social Epistemology Review & Reply Collective*, *4*(8), 66-75.

Kral, M. J. (1998). Suicide and the internalization of culture. *Transcultural Psychiatry*, *35*, 221-233.

Kral, M. J. & White, J. (2017). Moving toward a critical suicidology. *Annals of Psychiatry & Mental Health*, *5*(2), 1099.

Lester, D. (1972). *Why people kill themselves*. Springfield, IL: Charles Thomas/.

Lester, D. (1989). The study of suicide from a feminist perspective. *Crisis*, *11*, 38-43.

Lester, D. (1990). Suicide as a political act. *Psychological Reports*, *66*, 1185-1186.

Lester, D. (1997). The sexual politics of double suicide. *Feminism & Psychology*, *7*, 148-154.

Lester, D. (2003). *Fixin' to die*. Amityville, NY: Baywood.

Lester, D. (2004). *Katie's diary*. New York: Brunner-Routledge.

Lester, D. (2010). Female suicide bombers and burdensomeness. *Psychological Reports*, *106*, 160-162.

Lester, D. (2011). Female suicide bombers. *Suicidology Online*, *2*, 62-66.

Lester, D. (2014a). Oppression and suicide. *Suicidology Online*, *5*, 59-73.

Lester, D. (2014b). *The "I" of the storm*. Berlin, Germany: De Gruyter.

Lester, D. (2014c). *Rational suicide: Is it possible?* Hauppauge, NY: Nova Science.

Lester, D., McSwain, S. & Gunn, J. (2013). Suicide and the Internet: the case of Amanda Todd. *Journal of Emergency Mental Health & Human Resilience*, *15*(2-3), 179-180

Lester, D. & Stack, S. (2015). *Suicide as a dramatic performance*. New Brunswick, NJ: Transaction.

Marsh, I. (2010). *Suicide, Foucault, history and truth*. Cambridge, UK: Cambridge University Press.

Marsh, I. (2014, August 5). Suicide: the hidden cost of the financial crisis. *New Statesman*.

Peck, M. L. (1965). *The relation of suicidal behavior to characteristics of the significant other*. Ph.D. dissertation. University of Portland.

Pennebaker, J. W. & Stone, L. D. (2004). What was she trying to say? In D. Lester (Ed.) *Katie's diary*, pp. 55-79. New York: Brunner-Routledge.

Richman, J. (1986). *Family therapy for suicidal people*. New York: Springer.

Szasz, T. (1986). The case against suicide prevention. *American Psychologist*, *41*, 806-812.

White, J. (2012). Youth suicide as a 'wild problem:' Implications for prevention practice. *Suicidology Online*, *3*, 42-50.

White, J. (2015). Shaking up Suicidology. *Social Epistemology*, *4*(6), 1-4.

White, J. & Kral, M. (2014). Re-thinking youth suicide: Language, culture and power. *Journal of Social Action for Counseling and Psychology*, *6*(1), 122-142.

White, J., Marsh, I., Kral, M. J. & Morris, K. (2016). *Critical suicidology*. Vancouver, Canada: University of British Columbia.

In: The End of Suicidology
Editor: David Lester
ISBN: 978-1-53615-310-1


*Chapter 3*

# JOINER AND RUDD: EXPANDING THE BOUNDARIES

***David Lester, PhD***
Stockton University, Galloway, New Jersey, US

Joiner and Rudd (2000) edited a book on suicidology in which, in their own words, sought to expand the boundaries of the discipline. After two introductory chapters, the book contained 14 chapters which sought to do this.

Abramson, et al. (2000) reviewed some research on Beck's hopelessness theory of suicide (Beck et al., 1985) and proposed a process in which negative life events combine with a negative cognitive style to result in hopelessness and then, subsequently, to suicidality. The negative cognitive style involves attributing negative events to stable, global causes, viewing these events as very important, inferring that current negative events will lead to further negative consequences, and inferring that these negative events means that they themselves are flawed, unworthy or deficient in some way (Abramson, et al., 2000, p. 22). Abramson et al. also suggested the origins in childhood of the development of this negative cognitive style, such as parental psychopathology and early maltreatment (physical and emotional abuse).

Vohs and Baumeister (2000) developed Baumeister's escape theory of suicide in which suicidal behavior is an attempt to escape from painful self-awareness. Escape theory begins with people falling short of their goals and expectations and holding themselves responsible (self-blame). Along with hopelessness for the future, intense negative affect is generated from which the people desire to escape. Unable to generate appropriate cognitive strategies, they are more likely to consider suicide as an option. In this later paper, Vohs and Baumeister tied self-regulation into the theory. Self-regulation involves setting goals, changing the self so as to achieve those goals, and making the effort to achieve the goals. Thus, a failure in self-regulation can be seen as preceding the processes involved in the escape theory of suicide.

Cornette, et al. (2000) reviewed the theory presented in their earlier chapter (Abramson, et al., 2000), and add brief reviews of escape theory and self-discrepancy theory.[1] They discussed whether all three theories have potential for understanding suicide, and they also proposed that these theories may mean that that there are subtypes of suicidal individuals, with some fitting one theory better than the others. They also discussed whether it is possible to merge the theories and concluded that they can be integrated into a single theory.

Hastings, et al. (2000) reviewed research on the role of shame in motivating suicidal behavior, a variable that has often been associated with suicide in past scholarly articles (e.g., Lester, 1997). Catanzaro (2000) reviewed research on the role of mood regulation in suicidal behavior, a variable which has been noted in previous research (e.g., Williams & Pollock, 1993). Schmidt and Bates (2000) reviewed research on the incidence of suicidal behavior in patients with panic disorder and presented some new data on the topic. Riskind, et al. (2000) discussed what they call *looming vulnerability* and the precipitation of suicide. Looming vulnerability is when, faced with rapid, aversive changes (and stressful

[1] Self-discrepancy focuses on the conflicts between the ideal self, the ought self and actual self.

events), people experience strong and acute anxiety. De Leo (2010) has documented the presence of this in his interviews with survivors of serious attempts at suicide.

Verona and Patrick (2000) reviewed the evidence linking suicidal behavior to externalizing syndromes (such as reactive aggressiveness, persistent criminality, antisocial personality disorder and alcohol use disorders). These individuals are at risk for suicide because they are highly stress-reactive and prone to act impulsively. Davila and Daley (2000) discussed the role of interpersonal variables in suicidal behavior. Finally, Sachs-Ericsson (2000) discussed the role of gender and Young, et al. (2000) discussed the role of ethnicity.

## COMMENT

All of the chapters in Joiner and Rudd's book present excellent reviews of the topic chosen. However, they focus on variables that have been studied before for their association with suicidal behavior, although some (such as shame and looming vulnerability) have not received as much attention as other variables (such as hopelessness). Some of the chapters do present interesting flow charts for the development of suicidal behavior, but none present novel theories about suicide or provocative ideas.

## REFERENCES

Abramson, L. Y., Alloy, L. B., Hogan, M. E., Whitehouse, W. G., Gibb, B. E., Hankin, B. L. & Cornette, M. M. (2000). The hopelessness theory of suicidality. In T. Joiner & M. D. Rudd (Eds.) *Suicide science*, pp. 17-32. Boston, MA: Kluwer Academic.

Beck, A. T., Steer, R. a., Kovacs, M. & Garrison, R. (1985). Hopelessness and eventual suicide. *American Journal of Psychiatry*, *142*, 559-563.

Catanzaro, S. J. (2000). Mood regulation and suicidal behavior. In T. Joiner & M. D. Rudd (Eds.) *Suicide science*, pp. 81-103. Boston, MA: Kluwer Academic.

Cornette, M. M., Abramson, L. Y. & Bardone, A. M. (2000). Toward an integrated theory of suicidal behaviors. In T. Joiner & M. D. Rudd (Eds.) *Suicide science*, pp. 43-66. Boston, MA: Kluwer Academic.

Davila, J. & Daley, S. E. (2000). Studying interpersonal factors in suicide. In T. Joiner & M. D. Rudd (Eds.) *Suicide science*, pp. 175-200. Boston, MA: Kluwer Academic.

De Leo, D. (2010). *Turning points*. Bowen Hills, Australia: Australian Academic Press.

Hastings, M. E., Northman, L. M. & Tangney, J. P. (2000). Shame, guilt, and suicide. In T. Joiner & M. D. Rudd (Eds.) *Suicide science*, pp. 67-79. Boston, MA: Kluwer Academic.

Joiner, T. & Rudd, M. D. (2000). *Suicide science: Expanding the boundaries*. Boston, MA: Kluwer Academic.

Lester, D. (1997). The role of shame in suicide. *Suicide & Life-Threatening Behavior*, *27*, 352-361.

Riskind, J. H., Long, D. G., Williams, N. L. & White, J. C. (2000). Desperate acts for desperate times. In T. Joiner & M. D. Rudd (Eds.) *Suicide science*, pp. 105-115. Boston, MA: Kluwer Academic.

Sachs-Ericsson, N. (2000). Gender, social roles, and suicidal ideation and attempts in a general population sample. In T. Joiner & M. D. Rudd (Eds.) *Suicide science*, pp. 117-136. Boston, MA: Kluwer Academic.

Schmidt, N. B. & Bates, M. (2000). Suicide and panic disorder. In T. Joiner & M. D. Rudd (Eds.) *Suicide science*, pp. 201-220. Boston, MA: Kluwer Academic.

Verona, E. & Patrick, C. J. (2000). Suicide risk in externalizing syndromes. In T. Joiner & M. D. Rudd (Eds.) *Suicide science*, pp. 137-173. Boston, MA: Kluwer Academic.

Vohs, K. D. & Baumeister, R. F. (2000). Escaping the self-consumes regulatory resources. In T. Joiner & M. D. Rudd (Eds.) *Suicide science*, pp. 33-41. Boston, MA: Kluwer Academic.

Williams, J. M. G. & Pollock, L. R. (1993). Factors mediating suicidal behavior. *Journal of Mental Health*, *2*, 3-27.

Young, S., Twomey, H. & Kaslow, N. J. (2000). Suicidal behavior in African American women with a history of childhood maltreatment. In T. Joiner & M. D. Rudd (Eds.) *Suicide science*, pp. 221-240. Boston, MA: Kluwer Academic.

In: The End of Suicidology
Editor: David Lester
ISBN: 978-1-53615-310-1


*Chapter 4*

# Rogers and Lester: Proposals for the Future of Suicidology

***David Lester, PhD***
Stockton University, Galloway, New Jersey, US

Rogers and Lester (2010) in their co-authored book attempted to provide the groundwork for a new beginning for suicidology. They acknowledged that suicidology had seemed to have reached a dead end, but they had hope that this was only temporary. They examined methodological issues in suicide research, research in four disciplines (psychology, psychiatry, sociology and anthropology) and eight areas of research such as studies of sexual abuse and suicidality and studies of the suicidal personality. What was novel in the book was that each chapter concluded with *recommendations* for the future. Thus, they did not propose new theories, but rather suggested directions for future research and theorizing. For a full report, readers must read the original book, but I will present an example here from the chapter on typologies.

That chapter on typologies noted that samples of suicides appear to be composed of very heterogenous individuals. It may, therefore, be impossible to find a single theory of suicide that accounts for all of their suicidal acts.

They reviewed previous typologies such as that of Durkheim (1897) who defined anomic, altruistic, fatalistic and egoistic suicide, and an excellent piece of research by Reynolds and Berman (1995) which applied ten typologies to 484 cases of suicide whose information was obtained from the files of medical examiners. Rogers and Lester then made five recommendations for the future of research on typologies.

> *Recommendation 14.1:* It is important to develop meaningful psychology-based typologies of suicidal individuals.
>
> *Recommendation 14.2:* In order to bring suicidal behavior into mainstream psychology, it is important to develop typologies of suicidal behavior that are based on the classic theories of personality (or on theories from other fields in psychology).
>
> *Recommendation 14.3:* Although it is easier to develop empirically-based typologies of living suicidal individuals (such as suicide attempters and ideators), it is important to develop empirically-based typologies of completed suicides.
>
> *Recommendation 14.4:* "Arm-chair" typologies should be explored for their usefulness in generating hypotheses for research in order to identify those that are useful for increasing our understanding of suicide.
>
> *Recommendation 14.5:* Typologies of non-fatal suicidal behavior (attempts and ideation) should be explored for their usefulness in generating research that increases our understanding of suicidal behavior, in predicting short-term and long-term outcomes, and in formulating psychotherapeutic plans.

To illustrate the recommendations made for a discipline. Rogers and Lester made ten recommendations for anthropology, a discipline smaller in the number of scholars and one which has not made suicidal behavior a major focus. Indeed, the major theory proposed by an anthropologist was by Raoul Naroll in a book oddly entitled *Data Quality Control.*

> *Recommendation 6.1:* Anthropologists should devote more thought and research to the topic of suicidal behavior than they do at the present time.
>
> *Recommendation 6.2:* Anthropologists should identify and document the definitions of suicide in different cultures.
>
> *Recommendation 6.3:* Anthropologists should document the *meanings* and psychodynamics of suicidal behavior in different cultures.

*Recommendation 6.4:* Anthropologists should document the phenomenon of suicidal behavior in cultures to identify which aspects of the phenomenon are culture specific and which are found across all cultures.

*Recommendation 6.5:* Anthropological research should focus on the role of cultural conflict in suicidal behavior and the effect of different styles of coping with the conflict on suicidal behavior.

*Recommendation 6.6:* Anthropologists should endeavor to devise theories of suicide based on their studies of cultures rather than attempt to fit anthropological data within psychological and sociological theories.

*Recommendation 6.7:* Anthropologists should study suicidal behavior in the different ethnic groups within developed nations, groups which have been ignored by suicidologists hitherto.

*Recommendation 6.8:* Anthropologists should endeavor in their research to identify which aspects of suicidal behavior are (relatively) culturally invariant and which vary with culture.

*Recommendation 6.9:* The entries for suicide for all cultures in the Human Relations Area Files need to be gathered together, rated by independent judges so that inter-judge reliability can be assessed, specified by era, and explored for cross-cultural correlates.

*Recommendation 6.10:* Anthropologists should explore indigenous cultures for their theories of suicide and endeavor to test these theories empirically.

The number of recommendations for each chapter ranged from 4 to 18, and there a total of 105 recommendations. However, as noted above, Rogers and Lester did not propose any new theories of suicide.

## References

Durkheim, E. (1897). *Le suicide* [*Suicide*]. Paris, France, Felix Alcan.

Naroll, R. (1962). *Data quality control*: a *new research technique; prolegomena to a cross-cultural study of culture stress.* Glencoe, IL: Glencoe Free Press.

Reynolds, F. M. T. & Berman, A. L. (1995). An empirical typology of suicide. *Archives of Suicide Research*, *1*, 97-109.

Rogers, J. R. & Lester, D. (2010). *Understanding suicide: why we don't and how we might.* Cambridge, MA: Hogrefe.

# Provocative Ideas

In this section, I will present some ideas that may provoke creative thinking about suicidal behavior and suggest new theories of suicide.

In: The End of Suicidology
Editor: David Lester
ISBN: 978-1-53615-310-1


*Chapter 5*

# Brian Mishara's Two Component Model of Suicide with Life and Suicide Tendencies

***David Lester, PhD***
Stockton University, Galloway, New Jersey, US

Mishara (1996) noted that suicidologists (and psychologists in general) tended to seek relatively simple laws and theories to explain human behavior. Developmental psychologists, in particular, "attempt to control sufficient numbers of variables in order to isolate a few important factors that influence developmental processes" (p. 182). In contrast, physicists, among others, have developed techniques to study complex structures in open systems (e.g., Prigogine, 1980).

> These models challenge the simple and orderly world of Newtonian physics by examining structures whose determinants involve such complex and multivariate dimensions that the nature of their developmental changes over time can only be depicted after extensive and elaborate computer calculations. (Mishara, 1996, p. 182).

Mishara considered what seems paradoxical in that suicidal tendencies often have discontinuities over time. The desire to die by suicide can vary tremendously over time, over hours and minutes, and perhaps days and weeks. Mishara noted that research aimed at identifying the events and variables that predict suicidal behavior has failed. Mishra cited Pokorny's (1993) study of 4,800 consecutively admitted psychiatric patients which failed to find predictive factors for suicide using multivariate analyses.

Suicidal behavior develops over time but, although suicide is always an option, there are no events that are necessary or sufficient to precipitate suicidal behavior. Mishara proposed applying the ideas of Prigogine and others who study open systems interacting with complex environments, resulting sometimes in steady states, but at other times instabilities that result in complete reorganizations of the structure of the system.

To illustrate this idea, Mishara proposed the existence of two basic tendencies that vary over time: (i) a suicidal tendency D and (ii) a life tendency L. It could be, of course, that these two tendencies are merely opposite ends of a single dimension, but Mishara opted to view them as two separate tendencies.[1] These two tendencies can influence each other through a process of mutual inhibition, and this inhibition can be weak, moderate or strong. There are many experiences that can influence D, the suicidal tendency, such as loss of a partner or a diagnosis of a terminal disease. There are also many experiences that can affect L, the life tendency, such as falling in love or achieving a goal. The sum totals of all of these two sets of events can be labelled $S_D$ and $S_L$. The mutual inhibition of D and L is indicated by a parameter $\alpha$. This results in a model that describes changes over time of D and L using two equations.

$$dD/dt = -D + S_D - \alpha f(L) \qquad (1)$$

$$dL/dt = -L + S_L - \alpha f(D) \qquad (2)$$

[1] There is a parallel her, of course, with Freud's life and death instincts – Eros and Thanatos.

where dD/dt and dL/dt represent changes in the D and L tendencies over time. The functions f(L) and f(D) are unspecified, and it is not clear to me (DL) why D and L have minus signs.

Mishara proposed that, when alpha ($\alpha$) is weak, the two tendencies do not inhibit each other much, and there is one stable steady state in which suicidal and life tendencies co-exist. If alpha is a little larger (say $\alpha > 1$), then the steady state is unstable. Mishara suggested that this may occur in individuals with extreme psychopathologies and in those who are chronically suicidal and make multiple suicide attempts, for whom both suicidal and life tendencies are strong. As alpha gets larger, again there is one steady state and no unstable states. Mishara suggested that bipolar individuals fit this condition. When the individual is in a manic or a depressive state, these states tend to be stable and not influenced much by events.

It is only when alpha is large (say $\alpha > 2$), that it is possible to have two stable states and one unstable state. Slight changes in either D or L around this steady state result in increases in D and L, and there can be dramatic increases in the suicidal tendency. A family argument can increase the suicidal tendency (D) to crisis proportions, while a compassionate telephone call from a friend can increase the life tendency (L) and reverse the process. Mishara concluded, however, that predicting the suicidal behavior of an individual in this situation is very difficult.

## RATIONALITY VERSUS IRRATIONALITY

Bijou Yang Lester (Lester, B.Y., 2011), a behavioral economist, was interested in explaining the choices made by individuals. She proposed that choices are determined by a two-process model, with the individual's behavior affected by a rational component and an irrational component. Lester proposed a two-way cross-embedment model, which is similar to some extent to Mishara's idea of the D and L tendencies mutually influencing each other.

Lester's model distinguished between the components in the mind (such as thoughts) and the behavior. She noted that one can behave rationally or irrationally. However, when one behaves rationally, there may be irrational components, and, when one behaves irrationally, there may be rational components. Lester gave the example of credit card use. Carrying a zero balance and getting the cash bonus is rational behavior with a rational component. Carrying a non-zero balance but getting the cash bonus is irrational behavior with a rational component. Having a zero balance but no cash bonus is rational behavior with an irrational component. Carrying a non-zero balance and getting no cash bonus is irrational behavior with an irrational component.

Lester noted that two process (and, we might add, two tendency) models have some similarity to two-self models of the mind. In these models, there seem to be two (or more) subselves arguing with each other, struggling to make sense of the situation, and arriving at a decision. Lester (2015b) has proposed a multiple self theory of the mind, but he did not apply his model to suicidal behavior.

When individuals plan and stage their suicidal action, they have to make many choices, choices which will affect the likelihood of dying from the method chosen and the likelihood of others intervening and saving the individual (Lester, 2015a; Lester & Stack, 2015). For example, an individual planning suicide using an overdose can choose to take the overdose at home or in a motel away from home, and they can also vary the time of the evening and night when they consume the overdose, decisions that affect the chances of someone intervening to prevent the suicide. These choices are associated with the personal characteristics of the individuals (Lester & Stack, 2015), and some choices may be more rational than others or, in the present context, have rational and irrational components. For example, taking a lethal overdose (rational for dying by suicide) at home when other residents are likely to arrive home soon (irrational for dying by suicide) has both components.

## Discussion

The notion of two (and perhaps) more components which interact with one another in a decision leads to more complex theories than simple additive models, in which risk factors are weighted and summed to predict suicidal behavior. However, these two-component theories are in their early stages at the present time. More theoretical work needs to be done, and empirical tests of theories devised.

## References

Lester, B. Y. (2011). An exploratory analysis of composite choices. *Journal of Socio-Economics*, *40*, 949-958.

Lester, D. (2015a). Suicide as a staged performance. *Comprehensive Psychology*, *4*, #18.

Lester, D. (2015b). *On multiple selves*. New Brunswick, NJ: Transaction.

Lester, D. & Stack, S. (2015). *Suicide as a dramatic performance*. New Brunswick, NJ: Transaction

Mishara, B. L. (1996). A dynamic developmental model of suicide. *Human Development*, *39*, 181-194.

Pokorny, A. D. (1993). Suicide prediction revisited. *Suicide & Life-Threatening Behavior*, *23*, 1-10.

Prigogine, I. (1990). *From being to becoming*. San Francisco: Freeman.

In: The End of Suicidology
Editor: David Lester
ISBN: 978-1-53615-310-1


*Chapter 6*

# MEMES AND SUICIDE[1]

***David Lester, PhD***
Stockton University, Galloway, New Jersey, US

Dawkins (1976) developed the concept of *memes* to describe the cultural transmission of ideas, hoping to incorporate the process of evolution in a way which parallels genetic transmission and Darwinian evolution. The *evolution* of language is one example of the type of transmission in which Dawkins was interested. There are fashions and fads in "dress and diet, ceremonies and customs, art and architecture, engineering and technology" (p. 204) that also illustrate the concept

The word meme was defined as a unit of cultural transmission or unit of imitation. Dawkins chose this term because the Greek word mimeme means imitation. Examples of memes are "tunes, ideas, catch-phrases, clothing fashions, ways of making pots or of building arches" (p. 206). Heylighen (1992) defined a meme as an information pattern held in an individual's memory which is capable of being copied to another person's memory.

---

[1] This chapter is based on Lester (2009).

Using the analogy of genes and cells, Dawkins proposed that memes can be self-copying, that is, they can replicate.[2] The best memes, from an evolutionary point of view, must have longevity, fecundity, and copying-fidelity. Longevity refers to the length of time a meme can survive in time in a culture. Fecundity refers to how acceptable it is to the population. Copying-fidelity refers to the extent to which it remains unchanged in content as it is transmitted throughout cultures. Dawkins noted that copying-fidelity was probably rare since memes most likely continually mutate and blend with other memes.[3]

Dawkins asked that, if a tune was a meme, what is a symphony? He suggested that individual memes can combine into *meme complexes.* Individual memes can also become associated with other memes and be mutually assisting. Dawkins called these *co-adapted meme-complexes*.[4] Individual memes also compete for attention, because human minds are limited in capacity.

## Properties of Memes

Memes can spread fast, in a matter of hours, especially in this era of the Internet (Heylighen, 1992). This fast transmission to large numbers of people also increases the likelihood of mutation of memes, in the same way that rumors have been documented to change as they are passed from one individual to another. It is possible to talk of the evolution of memes, both (i) the gradual changing of a meme over time and (ii) the elimination of some memes from the culture while others survive. The memes best able to survive will be those with the best communicability.

The survival of memes depends on how simple and explicit they are as well as the genetic and cultural predispositions to learn them (Heylighen,

[2] *Replicate* is a more appropriate term than *self-copying* since memes require individuals and a society to replicate.

[3] Dawkins used the concepts of infection and also, at other times, viruses which, I think, introduce an unwelcome value judgment into what should be a neutral concept.

[4] Dawkins gave as an example here the God meme becoming associated with a hell-fire meme, the faith meme and, depending on the religion, memes affecting the lifestyle of individual.

1992). The most enduring memes are probably those which are consistent with genetic behavioral patterns. New memes which contradict previous memes will catch on less easily in a culture because people will tend to avoid cognitive dissonance (Festinger, 1957). Heylighen (1992) noted that some memes are more *contagious* than others, although it is not easy *a priori* to specify which memes will be more contagious and which will be less contagious. Finally, Heylighen noted that memes have the implicit goal of making their carriers more fit. This does not mean that the less fit members of a society will die (as in Darwinian evolution) for, unlike genes, memes as ideas easily survive the death of an individual who holds them.

Successful memes, Heylighen suggested, must be distinctive so that they will be noticed and assimilated. They should be novel, simple, coherent, and possess utility. Memes which come from accepted authority figures are precise and unambiguous and, reinforced by several individuals, will also be more likely to be successful. Memes which are beneficial only to their hosts will not necessarily survive. Successful memes are those which replicate more effectively. Memes can be stable and penetrating or, alternatively, transient and localized.

It should be noted that it is generally believed that the gene is not subjected to Darwinian evolution but rather it is the phenotype that is so subjected. The gene is the set of instructors (the replicator), whereas the phenotype is the physical manifestation. Memes are analogous to phenotypes, not genotypes, and so they are the result of instructions. Dawkins corrected this in a subsequent book (Dawkins, 1981), and what Dawkins originally called memes are more properly called *meme products*.

McGrath (2005) noted that the idea of memes was not original to Dawkins. Campbell (1960, 1988) introduced the idea of a "cultural replicator" which he called the mnemone in 1960; sociobiologists have introduced the concept of culturgen (Lumsden & Wilson, 1981); and Cloak (1975) proposed that culture evolves by means of a Darwinian mechanism. McGrath (2005) raised the critical question of whether memes actually exist. What is the evidence for memes, and what criteria can be proposed for their usefulness? McGrath noted that memes are *hypothetical constructs*, inferred from observation rather than observed themselves. McGrath argued that the construct of memes may not be as useful in the sense of generating hypotheses as is the use of the concept of simple cultural transmission.

## Archetypes and Memes

Several scholars have noted the similarity between memes and Jungian archetypes in the collective unconscious. The major difference, of course, is that memes are passed on via interpersonal and cultural transmission, whereas archetypes, as conceived by Jung, are inherited. Lester (1996) discussed what possible archetypes for suicide might be proposed, and so his discussion is relevant to suggesting possible memes for suicide. Specifically, Lester suggested that some types of suicide might be representative of archetypes. The kamikaze pilots of Japan in the Second World War aimed their planes at American ships or other targets and died in the subsequent crashes. They committed suicide for a cause, a heroic self-sacrifice. During the Iran–Iraq war, young Iranian soldiers performed similar sacrificial acts. In fact, in any war, soldiers give their lives to save fellow soldiers or civilians, as do firefighters and others involved in rescues on a daily basis. Although the story of Jesus's life may illustrate many archetypes, his reluctance to act so as to prevent his own death sentence and execution could be seen as similar, for he died willingly to save others. This theme of suicide as self-sacrifice occurs in daydreams and stories and perhaps reflects an archetype.

The Romeo and Juliet story also has potential as an archetype. In this story of the love of two people which the society will not permit, the people are young, usually teenagers. (Would a Romeo and Juliet story have as much power were the people middle-aged?) Their parents will not let them meet and certainly not become lovers, and so they seek union in death. The same theme has been documented in real life recently in the young lovers jumping to their deaths into the volcano at Mount Mihara in Japan (Ellis & Allen, 1961).

Nunn (1998) has discussed the possible relation between archetypes and memes and suggested that the manifestation of archetypes in people's thoughts and behaviors is equivalent to a set of memes (or a meme complex) but adds the extra ingredient of *awareness*. Some archetypes involve only one meme (such as the Mandala), but others involve a meme complex (such as the Hero). Nunn also noted that archetypes may contain some *core memes* and, in addition, "a cloud of more mutable ones that vary from representation to representation" (p. 348).

## MEMES AND SUICIDE

Dawkins (1976) mentioned suicide only in connection with the sterile bees who sting honey-wasp invaders and die as a result, or the runts of litters who give up trying to stay alive (which benefits their litter mates). Dawkins saw these actions as forms of altruistic suicide. In an analogous manner, martyrs, kamikaze pilots, and suicidal terrorists give up their lives to facilitate the spread of a meme or rather a meme-complex (a religious, ideological, or national cause).

Much of the recent discussion of memes and suicide has focused on the role of suggestion and imitation. The work of Phillips (1974) and others about the rise in suicides after the newsworthy death of a celebrity suicide has intrigued meme theorists.[5] The fact that a celebrity suicide is followed by imitation suicides in the next few days is of interest as an example of a possible meme product. For example, Phillips (1974) noted that the suicide of Marilyn Monroe in 1962 was followed by 198 more suicides in the following month in America than would be expected on the basis of chance. However, probably no one chooses suicide today as a result of Monroe's death in 1962, although they may model themselves on celebrity suicides in general as a way of enhancing their memory. The specific meme and meme product (suicide after Marilyn Monroe's death) were, therefore, not very contagious and only short-term in their influence on suicide.

[5] Marsden, P. (undated). Operationising memetics: suicide, the Werther effect, and work of David P. Phillips. Accessed at http://pespmcl.vub.ac.be/Conf/Meme'ap/Marsden.html. March 19, 2007.

However, if the meme of imitating suicides by choosing suicide oneself is conceptualized as an abstract meme and meme product, then imitation of suicides has occurred in many nations and over the course of many centuries. Not only did many Europeans commit suicide after reading Goethe's novel, *The Sorrows of Young Werther*, over 200 years ago, but such clusters of suicides have been documented in other nations and eras, such as in Japan in the 1700s after audiences viewed suicides in kabuki plays (Krysinska & Lester, 2006).

Thus, it is important to distinguish between specific and abstract memes as well as short-term and long-term memes. Some of the archetypes proposed by Lester (1996) and mentioned above could be construed or interpreted as abstract and long-term memes. For example, heroic self-sacrifice in the course of a war or suicide for the sake of vengeance may be an abstract, long-term meme. Suicide bombing may be a specific meme that is bounded in time during the late 20th and early 21st centuries.

Long-term memes and meme products may generalize over regions or remain specific to particular regions. The methods used for suicide are often identified with specific countries and so can be considered to be localized memes. For example, "taking the pipe" or putting one's head into the gas stove (that is, using domestic coal gas) was a common method of suicide in England in the 20th Century, and it has been replaced in part by the use of car exhaust after England switched to natural gas for domestic use, as natural gas is less toxic than coal gas (Clarke & Lester, 1989). In Singapore and Hong Kong, jumping is common as a means of suicide (Lester, 1994), while guns are used by the majority of American suicides (Clarke & Lester, 1989).[6] The use of these methods is clearly affected by their availablility (Clarke & Lester, 1989), but the fact that the majority of suicides in an area uses them signifies that an imitation effect may be occurring too. Indeed, sometimes methods are associated with a race or a sex. Guns are viewed as a "masculine" method whereas overdoses are viewed as a "feminine" method of suicide in the United States. Culture-bound suicidal acts may also be

[6] Culture-specific methods of suicide may be localized memes, such as self-immolation by Buddhist monks or swallowing battery acid in Africa.

examples of localized memes, such as sati in India and seppuku in Japan (Lester, 2004).

In contrast, it has long been known by members of societies that men complete suicide at a higher rate than women, whereas women attempt suicide (and survive) at a higher rate than men in the majority of societies (Lester, 1984). This difference has been reported in most eras and in most cultures and has become perhaps a societal expectation and self-fulfilling prophecy. Thus, it may represent a *long-term, generalized* meme. The spate of suicides after a celebrity suicide is a short-term meme, whereas the increased likelihood of suicide among elderly persons to avoid being a burden on the younger generations may be a long-term meme.

In earlier eras, memes were passed on in folk tales and stories, initially via verbal transmission (storytelling and performance) and later in books. Today, the advent of the Internet has speeded up the transmission of information, so that memes can spread quite rapidly. Information on methods for committing suicide is available on the web, as well as information on crisis intervention services to help prevent suicide (Lester, 2003). Strangers can contact one another to form suicide pacts, meeting to die by suicide together (Samuels, 2007). Others commit suicide while recording their acts on a video-cam which is transmitted to the Internet. It is possible, therefore, to claim that some suicide memes are prolific and "infect" many others rapidly. However, most memes remain localized and are only short-term. It is of interest to explore which memes generalize across cultures and which become embedded in a single culture.

Governments and others have tried to censor memes. Parents can restrict the websites to which their children have access. Governments have banned books on how to commit suicide, for example, in France (Soubrier, 1992), while other governments have criminalized the act of suicide (Lester, 2002) and religions conceptualize it as a sin (Lester, 2003).

Marsden (2000) noted that those who commit suicide typically have a reduced capacity to pass on ideas. Suicidal individuals tend to be socially isolated, socially disenfranchised, and labelled as deviants (and thereby devalued by the culture) [7]. Suicide, "spreading by infection over the media, could be tolerated within a culture as long as it affected those with neutral or negative sociocultural inclusive reproductive potential" (Marsden, 2000, p. 99). On the other hand, altruistic suicide may enhance the status and prestige of the individual, and this may in turn increase the likelihood of the suicide meme being passed on.

The transmission of memes raises the issue of which members of a culture are susceptible to, not just a particular meme (such as, for example, the Romeo and Juliet meme[8]), but also the meme product, that is, actually choosing suicide as a result of a love which cannot be consummated. Which individuals in the culture are susceptible to modelling, especially modelling behavior that is frowned upon and which requires *disinhibitory contagion* (Marsden, 2000) in order for the individual to engage in the behavior. Hearing of an individual who has committed suicide may be sufficient to resolve internal conflicts about whether to engage in that behavior. Observing a representation of suicide may reduce internal restraints against suicide, that is, it may result in disinhibition.

Marsden (2000) suggested that, in modelling, an individual in distress who chooses between a suicidal or a nonsuicidal solution may look at how others have resolved similar problems. If others, especially others with high prestige, have chosen suicide, then this may reinforce that particular choice. Whereas modelling is a conscious process, *priming* is a relatively involuntary aspect of social cognition. Marsden also suggested that priming in general may be an inherited cognitive mechanism that increases the chance of survival. The information obtained by observing other members of the species can be a valuable resource which may be used in a relatively automatic way to guide the behavior of the observer. In the case of suicide, however, priming results in the destruction of the individual, but perhaps

---

[7] This statement parallels the argument made by sociobiologists that those who die by suicide are persons who are less likely to pass on their genes to future generations, such as the elderly and the childless (DeCatanzaro, 1981).

[8] The Romeo and Juliet theme is more likely a meme-complex with many components which makes suicide is such situations more likely.

this occurs only for those who are distressed and susceptible to self-destructive actions in the first place. Range, Goggin, and Steede (1988) gave students a vignette of a distressed individual to read. Some were told that this individual knew someone who had died by suicide (priming), while others were not given this information. The mention of suicide in the vignette increased the estimate of the probability that the students would choose suicide under a similar circumstance, indicating that priming changed the students' responses. It would be unethical, of course, to conduct a priming experiment in which one investigated which individuals might actually commit suicide.

## CONCLUSION

This chapter has explored contributions of the concept of memes to the study of suicide. The concept of memes stimulates exploration of the ideas, themes, and myths about suicide that exist in various cultures. Examples were given that cultures differ in preferred methods for suicide, have different acceptable motives for suicide, and differ in myths held about suicide (such as that completed suicide is a masculine behavior, while attempted suicide is a feminine behavior).

The concept of memes can also be applied to the study of contagion, imitation, and modelling of suicidal behavior. Again, while not providing explanations for these phenomena, memetics[9] raises many questions which suicidologists have not considered hitherto, such as which suicide memes survive beyond a brief period of time (and why they survive), which ones spread from localized regions to broader regions (and eventually to whole cultures), and whether there could be both specific and abstract memes. Memetics may, therefore, provide a stimulus for suicidology

[9] The study of memes.

# REFERENCES

Campbell, D. T. (1960). Blind variation and selective retention in creative thought as in other knowledge processes. *Psychological Review*, *67*, 380-400.

Campbell, D. T. (1988). A general 'selection theory' as implemented in biological evolution and in social belief-transmission-with-modification in science. *Biology & Philosophy*, *3*, 171-177.

Clarke, R. V. & Lester, D. (1989). *Suicide: closing the exits*. New York: Springer-Verlag.

Cloak, F. T. (1975). Is a cultural ethology possible? *Human Ecology*, *31*, 161-182.

Dawkins, R. (1976). *The selfish gene*. New York: Oxford University Press.

Dawkins, R. (1981). *The extended phenotype*. Oxford, UK: Freeman.

DeCatanzaro, D. (1981). *Suicide and self-damaging behavior*. San Diego, CA: Academic Press.

Ellis, E. R. & Allen, G. N. (1961). *Traitor within*. Garden City, NY: Doubleday.

Festinger, L (1957). *A theory of cognitive dissonance*. New York: Harper.

Heylighen, F. (1992). 'Selfish' memes and the evolution of cooperation. *Journal of Ideas*, *2*, 70-76.

Krysinska, K. & Lester, D. (2006). Comment on the Werther effect. *Crisis*, *27*, 10.

Lester, D. (1984). Suicide. In C. S. Widom (Ed.), *Sex roles and psychopathology*. New York: Plenum. Pp. 145-156.

Lester, D. (1994). Suicide by jumping in Singapore as a function of high-rise apartment availability. *Perceptual and Motor Skills*, *79*, 74.

Lester, D. (1996). Jungian perspectives on the unconscious and suicide. In A. A. Leenaars & D. Lester (Eds.), *Suicide and the unconscious*. Northvale, NJ: Jason Aronson. pp. 49-66.

Lester, D. (2002). Decriminalization of suicide in seven nations and suicide rates. *Psychological Reports*, *91*, 898.

Lester, D. (2003). *Fixin' to die*. Amityville, NY: Baywood.

Lester, D. (2004). *Thinking about suicide*. Hauppauge, NY: Nova Science.

Lester, D. (2009). Memes and suicide. *Psychological Reports*, *105*, 3-10.

Lumsden, C. J. & Wilson, E. O. (1981). *The coevolutionary process*. Cambridge, MA: Harvard University Press.

Marsden, P. (2000). *The 'Werther' effect: fact or fantasy?* Unpublished dissertation, University of Sussex, UK.

McGrath, A. (2005). *Dawkins' God*. Malden, MA: Blackwell.

Nunn, C. M. H. (1998). Archetypes and memes. *Journal of Consciousness Studies*, *5*, 344-354.

Phillips, D. P. (1974). The influence of suggestion on suicide. *American Sociological Review*, *39*, 340-354.

Range, L. M., Goggin, W. C. & Steede, K. K. (1988). Perception of behavioral contagion of suicide. *Suicide & Life-Threatening Behavior*, *18*, 334-341.

Samuels, D. (2007). Let's die together. *The Atlantic*, 299(4), 92-98.

Soubrier, J. P. (1992). From suicide prevention to suicide promotion. In D. Lester (Ed.), *Suicide '92*. Denver, CO: American Association of Suicidology., pp. 263-264.

In: The End of Suicidology
Editor: David Lester
ISBN: 978-1-53615-310-1


*Chapter 7*

# SUICIDE AS A STAGED PERFORMANCE[1]

***David Lester, PhD***
Stockton University, Galloway, New Jersey, US

Shakespeare, in his play *As You Like It*, said that "all the world's a stage, and all the men and women merely players." Nikolai Evreinov (1927), a Russian playwright and essayist, formalized this notion by arguing that we are theatrical beings and that everything that we do in our daily lives is a drama staged by ourselves, in his words a *monodrama*. If Evreinhov was correct, and everything in life is theatrical, why should our dying be anything less?

On September 18, 2010, Mitchell Heisman, aged 35, dressed himself in a white tuxedo, white tie, white shoes and white socks. He went to Harvard Yard, a green area on the Harvard University campus, and shot himself in the head with a silver revolver on the steps of the Memorial Church in front of a group of tourists. He left a 1,500-page suicide note online, with copies mailed to friends and family.[2]

---

[1] Adapted from Lester (2015a).

[2] For a discussion of this suicide note see Lester (2015b).

At 5 am on August 15, 2013, Martin Manley, aged 60, went to the parking lot of his local police station, called the officers inside, told them where he was and that he intended to shoot himself. He then shot himself. Manley had spent the last eighteen months creating a website outlining his life and the reasons for his decision to die by suicide. He chose the setting for his death in order to spare his landlord and siblings from having to discover his body.[3]

Not every suicidal death is as dramatic as these two examples, but it can be argued that every suicidal person stages their suicidal action. They make choices as to whether to leave a note, what method of suicide to use, what to wear, where to die, and whether they want witnesses to their action. Many of these decisions have personal meaning, but there are also gender and cultural scripts that affect people's choices. It is well documented that many suicides have made previous non-fatal suicidal acts and, in the present context, these non-fatal acts can be viewed as rehearsals for their later fatal action.

Dramatic performances typically involve a script, rehearsals, wardrobe, venue, audience, and the actual performance. Although dramatic performances often have a written script and an audience and take place in a theater, these elements are not necessary. For example, dramatic performances can be improvised and, therefore, lack a script. Dramatic performances construct a meaning through the selection of actions and arrangements. Most dramatic performances require a director, choreographer, lighting designer, sound designer, costume designer and set designer, but these roles may be played by one person.[4]

Rubenstein (2015) noted that the writings of Erving Goffman (1959) present a dramaturgical model of social life, and the role playing by the suicidal actor reminds us that individuals choosing suicide do so in relation to an audience. In the *performance*, a social message is conveyed. Whether the actor is aware of it or not, impression management is occurring, and the audience attributes meaning to the act. There is a setting with scenery, props, and location which are central to the performance. The protagonist is playing

---

[3] For a discussion of Manley's death and website, see Lester (2014a).

[4] http://dlibrary.acu.edu.au/faculties/learndrama/performance.htm.

a role, and we can consider whether the performance is consistent with what we know about the actor. Inconsistent performances require a more complex reading of the script.

The present chapter will discuss briefly these choices made by suicidal individuals when planning the staging of their suicidal act, what these choices tell us about these individuals, and what research needs to be done to help us better understand these choices.

## THE SUICIDE NOTE

A good proportion of suicides leave a suicide note, and this gives the individual an opportunity to present themselves to their significant others. For example, Haines, Williams and Lester (2011) found that 347 of 1051 consecutive suicides in Tasmania left a suicide note (33%). Yang and Lester (2011) argued that, contrary to the belief of suicidologists who conduct research on the suicidal mind by studying suicide notes, studies of suicides may not provide clues into the mind of the suicide since this *social self* which is presented to others may hide (or mask) the *real self* or *true self*.

As noted above, not all suicides leave a note. Why do some suicides leave notes while others do not? Some suicides notes read like last wills, and they give instructions to their significant others. Other suicide notes present reasons for the decision to die by suicide, and their significant others may find this helpful in resolving their grief. On the other hand, the suicide note can express anger toward the significant others. In contrast, the friends and relatives of those who do *not* leave a suicide notes often are obsessed with the question of why the individual chose to die by suicide. These choices made by the suicide have an impact on the significant others, and this impact may be chosen intentionally by the suicide.

The body can also be a "suicide note." If suicides die in such a way that significant others will find their body, they have left a "communication" in choosing this particular death scene. Finding the body leaves a lasting image in the minds of the significant others which increases the traumatic impact of the event, and this may have been the intent of the suicide. In rare cases, suicide notes have been written on the skin of the suicide (Austin & Byard, 2013). These may indicate loneliness and a lack of significant others or a lack of preparation and forethought.

These days suicide notes may appear in social media. The 1,500-page suicide note of Mitchell Heisman and the website created by Martin Manley were mentioned above. One 15-year-old girl in Canada posted a video on YouTube in which she silently displayed a sequence of flash cards detailing a history of bullying (Lester, 2015b). She posted the video on September 2 and died by suicide on October 10. The video received 1.6 million views, but, according to newspaper reports, no one intervened during that period.

An 18-year-old girl in Texas died by suicide after sending 145 tweets in the 24 hours prior to her death, detailing her experience of sexual abuse by her father and previous suicide attempts. During the series of tweets, there were two breaks (of 139 minutes and 21 minutes), yet no one intervened to stop her death. Interestingly, she made many of her tweets rhyme so that the tweets read like poems (Gunn & Lester, 2012).

Suicide notes using social media provide ample opportunity for intervention, but it is not known what proportion of suicides are prevented. We hear, instead, of those suicides for whom no one intervened.

## What to Wear

People have to make a choice as to what to wear when they die by suicide. The members of the Heaven's Gate cult, who died as a group in California in March 1976, all dressed exactly alike. They used phenobarbital dissolved in vodka and applesauce and pulled plastic bags over their heads. Their heads were shaved clean, and each had a five-dollar bill and three quarters (25 cents) in a pocket. They wore black shirts, sweat pants and Nike Decades athletic shoes. All had their face and torso covered with a square piece of black cloth. This uniformity of dress symbolized their membership in the group action.

Some suicides die naked (Simon, 2008), perhaps to symbolize rebirth and cleansing, to shock those who discover them, to be tidy or exhibitionistic, or simply because the method chosen for suicide demanded nakedness (such as drowning in a bathtub).

The mode of dress can be used to detect potential suicides. Gaylord and Lester (1994) noted that the Hong Kong subway system has surveillance cameras, and staff have identified clues that potential suicides show, including putting bags down as the train approaches the station (whereas regular passengers pick up their bags), standing by the wall where the train enters, hiding their faces with hats or scarves, and their choice of clothes. Prostitutes usually dress in an ornate red silk dress, while elderly Chinese wear traditional ethnic clothes. The staff who observe these clues are trained to approach the person and engage them in conversation, hoping to avert their suicide.

## WHICH METHOD TO USE

Each suicide must choose a method for their action. Clarke and Lester (2013) listed twenty possible influences for this choice:

1. Availability (e.g., owning a car)
2. Familiarity with the method (e.g., car exhaust gases)
3. Technical skills needed (hanging, gassing)
4. Planning necessary (buy a gun, save up drugs)
5. Likely pain (cutting wrists)
6. Courage needed (high building, train)
7. Consequences of failure (disability, publicity)
8. Disfigurement after death (hanging versus overdose)
9. Danger and inconvenience to others (car crash, subway leap)
10. Messiness and bloodiness (wrist cutting)
11. Discovery of body (by loved ones or strangers)
12. Contamination of nest (i.e., avoid home)

13. Scope for concealing or publicizing death-for the purposes of shaming others or insurance (car-crash, drowning, subway leap)
14. Certainty of death (perceived or actual)
15. Time taken to die while conscious (poisons, wrist cutting)
16. Scope for second thoughts (swim back to shore, switch off gas)
17. Chances of intervention ("fate," estranged lover)
18. Symbolism (cleansing by fire, seppuku)
19. Masculine/feminine (e.g., guns)
20. Dramatic impact (lover's leap versus overdose)

The most common explanation for the choice of method for suicide is convenience and accessibility of the method and, as a result, one tactic for preventing suicide has been to propose restricting access to lethal methods for suicide (Clarke & Lester, 2013), such as fencing in the bridges from which people jump and detoxifying the gas used in homes for heating and cooking.

There has been some research on simple personal characteristics that are associated with choice of method. For example, women generally choose less violent methods than do men. There are also ethnic differences with, for example, Asians and Asian-Americans choosing fire (self-immolation) more than other ethnic groups. However, what is perhaps more important is to identify the psychodynamic reasons for the choice of method. For example, Grumet (1989) reported the case of a male registered nurse, 35 years old and married, who took an overdose of imipramine and then connected a defibrillator to his head and released the electric charge through his brain. The man was a perfectionist and viewed himself as a failure. He frequently experienced guilt and depression. He also feared having a heart attack after suffering a mild heart attack at the age of 31. Grumet saw the choice of electricity as a symbolic way of execution for his sins (akin to convicted prisoners dying in the electric chair) and as a symbolic way of curing himself (akin to electroconvulsive therapy). Thus, the choice of method for suicide for this man had a very personal meaning.

## Where to Die

Suicides must make a choice of where to die: at home or away from home; in the presence of others or when isolated; if away from home, where (a hotel room, a national park); if home, in which room, etc.? Suicide when others are present provides an opportunity for bystanders (friends, relatives or strangers) to intervene. Steer, Beck, Garrison and Lester (1988) found that those attempted suicides who were interrupted during the act were much more likely to eventually die by suicide than were attempted suicides who attempted alone (14.6% versus 4.8%) and they died sooner (after 32 months versus 54 months). Bystanders do not always intervene to prevent the suicide from occurring. Cases have been reported of where strangers observing a potential suicide (such as an individual standing on a ledge about to jump) baited the individual and urged him to jump (Mann, 1981).

Suicide in public also shocks those witnessing the event. Bud Dwyer shot himself during a press conference in January 1987. He was the Treasurer for the state of Pennsylvania and about to be sentenced for bribery. Some reporters in the room ran for help, others tried to approach him, while others simply screamed and cursed. Several televisions stations showed the complete sequence. In July 1974, Christine Chubbuck, a television news reporter, shot herself on live television during the news broadcast. She said on camera: "In keeping with Channel 40's policy of bringing you the latest in blood and guns and in living color, you are going to see another first – attempted suicide." She then shot herself in the head and died. She had a history of depression, a recent romantic rejection, and had just been informed by her physician that she would have difficulty ever having a baby.

Stack (2015a) has explored the characteristics of those who choose to die in hotel room rather than at home, and those who choose a natural area (such as the Grand Canyon). In his study of those who travel away from home and who use a firearm, which Stack (2015b) called the Paladin pattern after the television series *Have Gun, Will Travel*, Stack found that men were twice as likely as women to follow this pattern, married individuals more likely than single individuals, and whites more than those of other ethnicities. The Paladin pattern was more common in those with a history of violence, but less common in those with psychiatric problems. The pattern was more common if the suicidal individual had used marijuana, but less common in opiate users and alcoholics.

Recently, Dogan, Demirci and Deniz (2015) examined 20 suicides in Konya, Turkey, who hung themselves from trees. These suicides comprised 11% of all the suicides by hanging and occurred primarily in the garden of the suicide's house (9 cases) and in woodlands (7 cases). All of these suicides lived in rural or small communities, and this method was used primarily by men (16 cases). Ten of the suicides (50%) occurred at night, and these ten all chose the garden of their home (9 cases) or the hospital in which they resided (1 case). The suicides during the daytime were more likely to travel to woodlands (by motor cycle or by foot), and Dogan, et al. suggested that this was to prevent intervention by others. (They noted one earlier case of a suicide by hanging in the woods who was found only after 29 years.) One of the suicides tied his hands together, presumably to prevent him changing his mind and attempting to abort the suicidal act. Dogan, et al. also suggested that, although the choice of method and location may be affected by convenience and access, the choice may also have symbolic meaning, noting that Judas Iscariot hung himself on a tree after betraying Jesus.

## Attempting Suicide as a Rehearsal

The single best predictor of subsequent suicide is a previous suicide attempt (Mann, 2002). Gunn (2015) cast attempted suicide as a rehearsal. His review of research found that, in general, those who used violent methods for the suicide attempt were more likely to repeat their suicidal behavior, both as attempted suicide and completed suicide. It is interesting that some suicides stay with one method, whereas others switch methods. There has been no research on the psychological differences between those who stay and those who switch.

Gunn noted that attempting suicide as a predictor for subsequent fatal suicidal behavior fits neatly into Joiner's (2005) Interpersonal Psychological

Theory of Suicide which proposes that an acquired capability for suicide is a prerequisite for suicide. Attempting suicide is one of the many experiences (such as combat experience or experience of physical and sexual abuse) which helps develop this capability.

## Cultural Scripts

There are cultural (and subcultural) scripts for suicidal acts, such as seppuku in Japan and sati in India. Culture can determine the location of the act and the method chosen. For example, in Tikopia in the South Pacific Ocean, the preferred methods are swimming out to sea and also strangling oneself by tying a rope around one's neck, securing it on a hook, and then running at high speed through the house (Firth, 1961). Interestingly, in this latter case, it is customary for the individuals to fast beforehand so that they do not soil themselves if they lose control of their bowels.

Among the subcultural scripts are suicidal acts such as victim-precipitated homicide, in which individuals provoke others into killing them, making the act seem to be one of murder rather than suicide, a method that Wolfgang (1958) found in Philadelphia to be more common among African Americans than among European Americans. The assumption is that, for these individuals, suicide is morally unacceptable whereas being killed by another is morally acceptable.

A variant of this is suicide-by-cop (Lindsay & Lester, 2004), in which individuals provoke police officers into killing them. Lindsay and Lester presented a series of clues that police officers might use to identify a potential suicide-by-cop incident.

- Incident initiated by subject
- Subject creates an event to ensure police response
- Subject forces confrontation
- Subject initiates aggressive action
- Presence of a deadly weapon
- Subject advances toward officer

- Subject refuses to drop weapon
- Retreat by officers
- Injured officer or citizen
- Subject threatens officer with a weapon

These clues constitute a script for this type of suicidal act.

## Discussion

Not every suicidal act is as dramatic as that of Mitchell Heisman mentioned in the introduction to this article. But every suicide has to make choices for the staging of the suicidal act. In making these choices, the suicides are deciding how they want to be viewed by others and how they want to be evaluated and remembered after their death. The choices that they make are determined, in part, by their psychodynamics and how they want to present themselves to others.

### The Need for Qualitative Research

There have been studies of some simple personal characteristics that are associated with the choices made by suicides, such as age, sex and ethnicity, but what is needed to further our understanding of these aspects of the suicidal act is qualitative research that explores the reasons behind the choices that suicides make. Of course, suicides are deceased and cannot be interviewed, but those who make near-fatal attempts at suicide, with strong suicidal intent, can be interviewed by psychodynamic-oriented clinicians. Qualitative research is not easy to carry out and sometimes difficult to get accepted by scholarly journals, but it would advance our understanding more than simplistic quantitative research does. A recent excellent example of this type of research appeared from De Leo (2010) who interviewed serious suicide attempters about their state of mind leading up to and immediately prior to their attempt. What was most interesting in their accounts was the presence of acute anxiety immediately prior to their attempt, a feature that has not received much attention in past research (Lester, 2014b).

## Impulsive Suicides

Some suicides appear to be impulsive and, for these suicides, the staging of the suicidal act may be minimal and the proposals made by the present chapter may less applicable. For example, Cheah, Schmitt and Pridmore (2008) reported the case of a young man who had misappropriated some money and lost it while gambling. He was crossing a bridge and, one-third of the way across, began to worry about being found out. He decided to kill himself and jumped from a height of forty-nine meters but survived. The psychiatrist who examined him afterwards found no evidence of Axis I or Axis II psychiatric disorders. The decision process for this young man, therefore, lasted only a few seconds. Studies of attempted suicides have reported that, for many, the decision process was brief. Simon, Swan, Powell, Potter, Kresnow and O"Carroll (2001) found that 24% of attempted suicides took less than five minutes between the decision to die by suicide and the actual act, and 5% just one second. Williams, Davidson and Montgomery (1980) reported that impulsive attempters were more often in the presence of others, thought that they would survive, were less depressed than non-impulsive attempters and experienced reduced tension as a result of the attempt. It is unknown what proportion of completed suicides is impulsive, although it is probably much less than the proportion of attempted suicides that is impulsive.

## Gender, Social and Cultural Scripts

This perspective of suicide as a dramatic act draws attention to the role of gender, social and cultural factors in the staging of suicide. It is well known that the methods used for suicide vary greatly from one society to another (Lester, 1990), but the staging of suicidal actions also varies greatly from one society to another, varying in such variables as location and clothes worn. Societies vary greatly in the role of conformity versus individualism (Triandis, 1993; Konsky, Eguchi, Blue & Kapoor, 1990), and members of the more conforming societies may have more similar scripts for their suicidal acts.

Furthermore, research has consistently shown that there are sex differences in the rate of suicide, the methods chosen, and other decisions, such as the location for the suicide. Stack (2015c) found that women in the United States in 2003-2006 were more likely to die by suicide at home than were men. Women are also more likely to attempt suicide and survive than are men while men die more often than do women (Lester, Gunn & Quinnett, 2014). The scripts chosen for suicidal acts may differ, therefore, for women and men.

## The Decision-Making Process

Although there is research on problem-solving behavior and decision-making choices in general in attempted suicides, the research utilizes tests of general problem-solving and has not explored the problem-solving and decision-making relevant to suicide. For example, Liu, Vassileva, Gonzalez and Martin (2012) compared attempted suicides and controls for whether they would accept $5 now versus $10 one week from now (a choice known as delay-discounting). The suicide attempters were more likely to choose the immediate reward. But this is *not* a study of the decision-making process involved in staging one's suicide.

The ideas presented in the present paper indicate that two decisions have to be made by the potential suicide. First, the individual has to decide to die by suicide, and then decide how to arrange this act. There is no research on these decisions, only clinical guesses by psychotherapists who have treated a particular suicidal individual and presented, in a case study, their speculations about the psychodynamics of the suicide. For example, in the case of Mitchell Heisman mentioned in the beginning, there are no clues in the newspaper reports of his suicide or in his 1,500-page suicide note as to why he dressed in white, why he chose a silver gun and why he chose the location of Harvard Yard.

Lester (1988a) reported a study which provides an example of the type of research that is needed. Lester studied the choice of method for suicide in a non-clinical population of 72 undergraduate students enrolled in a psychology course (and, therefore, most likely not suicidal). He asked them to consider, if they were going to die by suicide, would they use an overdose of pills or a gun. Nineteen chose a gun and 53 an overdose of pills. Those who choose pills rather than guns saw the use of pills as less quick, less painful, less planned and less "bad" (the term presented to the subjects). In a second study (of 429 undergraduates), Lester (1988b) found that women rated pain, disfigurement and the availability of the method as more important reasons for choosing a method for suicide than did men. These judgments about the methods of suicide most likely impact the method chosen by a suicidal individual.

These studies present subjects with dimensions (quick-slow, painful-painless) decided upon by the researcher. A better technique for the research would be to let the subjects choose their own dimensions with which to rate the methods for suicide using a technique similar to the Role Construct Repertory Grid technique devised by George Kelly (1955) for having subjects describe the significant others in their life. Of course, the research needs to be conducted on those who made serious attempts to die by suicide, but who survived, rather than non-suicidal undergraduates.

## Final Comment

Viewing suicide as a dramatic performance, in which individuals make conscious (or unconscious) choices as to how to stage their suicidal action, raises interesting questions about the psychodynamic reasons behind these choices. Viewing suicide from this perspective may also provide clues for the impending suicidal act, as in the cases of suicide-by-cop in the United States and suicide in ethnic Chinese individuals in the Hong Kong subway system noted earlier. If elements of cultural and subcultural scripts are observed by onlookers, intervention is possible. In addition, the choices (of location, methods, whether alcohol is consumed, dress, etc.) made by those who make attempts at suicide may have predictive value for future, fatal suicidal behavior. For example, Runeson, et al. (2010) found that those choosing hanging for their suicide attempt had the greatest likelihood of later dying by suicide.

Finally, I have argued that our understanding of the staging of suicidal acts may be advanced more by qualitative case studies rather than by quantitative research which tends to focus on distal variables rather than the psychodynamic factors affecting people's behavior.

## References

Austin, A. E. & Byard, R. W. (2013). Skin messages in suicide. *Journal of Forensic & Legal Medicine*, *20*, 618-620.

Cheah, D., Schmitt, S. & Pridmore, S. (2008). Suicide, misappropriation and impulsivity. *Australian & New Zealand Journal of Psychiatry*, *42*, 544-546.

Clarke, R. V. & Lester, D. (2013). *Suicide: closing the exits*. New Brunswick, NJ: Transaction.

De Leo, D. (2010). *Turning points*. Bowen Hills, Australia: Australian Academic Press.

Dogan, K. H., Demirci, S. & Deniz, I. (2015). Why do people hang themselves on trees? *Journal of Forensic Sciences*, *60*, (Supplement 1), S87-S92.

Evreinov, N. (1927). *The theatre in life*. New York: Benjamin Blom.

Firth, R. (1961). Suicide and risk-taking in Tikopia society. *Psychiatry*, *24*, 1-17.

Gaylord, M. S. & Lester, D. (1994). Suicide in the Hong Kong subway. *Social Science & Medicine*, *38*, 427-430.

Goffman, E. (1959). *The presentation of self in everyday life.* Garden City, NY: Doubleday.

Grumet, G. W. (1989). Attempted suicide by electrocution. *Bulletin of the Menninger Clinic*, *53*, 512-521.

Gunn, J. F. (2015). The rehearsal: non-fatal suicidal behavior as a precipitant of suicide. In D. Lester & S. Stack (Eds.), *Suicide as a dramatic performance*. New Brunswick, NJ: Transaction.

Gunn, J. F. & Lester, D. (2012). Twitter postings and suicide. *Suicidologi*, *17*(3), 28-30.

Haines, J., Williams, C. L. & Lester, D. (2011). The characteristics of those who do and do not leave suicide notes. *Omega*, *63*, 79-94.

Joiner, T. E. (2005). *Why people die by suicide*. Cambridge, MA: Harvard University Press.

Kelly, G. (1955). *The psychology of personal constructs*. New York: Norton.

Konsky, C., Eguchi, M., Blue, J. & Kapoor, S. (1999). Individualist-collectivist values. *Intercultural Communication Studies*, *9*(1), 69-82.

Lester, D. (1988a). The perception of different methods of suicide. *Journal of General Psychology*, *115*, 215-217.

Lester, D. (1988b). Why do people choose particular methods for suicide? *Activitas Nervosa Superior*, *30*, 312-314.

Lester, D. (1990). Changes in the methods used for suicide in 16 countries from 1960 to 1980. *Acta Psychiatrica Scandinavica*, *81*, 260-261.

Lester, D. (2014a). *Rational suicide, is it possible: reflections on the suicide of Martin Manley*. Hauppauge, NY: Nova Science.

Lester, D. (2014b). *The "I" of the storm*. Warsaw, Poland: De Gruyter.

Lester, D. (2015a). Suicide as a staged performance. *Comprehensive Psychology*, *4*, #18.

Lester, D. (2015b). Dramatic suicide notes. In D. Lester & S. Stack (Eds.), *Suicide as a dramatic performance*. New Brunswick, NJ: Transaction.

Lester, D., Gunn, J. F. & Quinnett, P. (2014). *Suicide in men*. Springfield, IL: Chares C. Thomas.

Lindsay, M. & Lester, D. (2004). *Suicide by cop*. Amityville, NY: Baywood.

Liu, R. T., Vassileva, J., Gonzalez, R. & Martin, E. M. (2012). A comparison of delay discounting among substances users with and without suicide attempt history. *Psychology of Addictive Behaviors*, *26*, 980-985.

Mann, J. J. (2002). A current perspective on suicide and attempted suicide. *Annals of Internal Medicine*, *136*, 302-311.

Mann, L. (1981). The baiting crowd in episodes of threatened suicide. *Journal of Personality & Social Psychology*, *41*, 703-709.

Rubenstein, J. (2015). Ritual, dramatic performance, and suicide. In D. Lester & S. Stack (Eds,), *Suicide as a dramatic performance*. New Brunswick, NJ: Transaction.

Runeson, B., Tidemalm, D., Dahlin, M., Lichtenstein, P. & Långström, N. (2010). Method of attempted suicide as predictor of subsequent successful suicide. *British Medical Journal*, *340*, c3222.

Simon, R. I. (2008). Naked suicide. *Journal of the American Academy of Psychiatry & the Law*, *36*, 240-245.

Simon, T. R., Swann, A. C., Powell, K. E., Potter, L. P., Kresnow, M. & O'Carroll, W. W. (2001). Characteristics of impulsive suicide attempts and attempters. *Suicide & Life-Threatening Behavior*, *32*(supplement), 49-59.

Stack, S. (2015a). The location of the suicidal act. In D. Lester & S. Stack (Eds.), *Suicide as a dramatic performance*. New Brunswick, NJ: Transaction.

Stack, S. (2015b). Have gun, will travel. In D. Lester & S. Stack (Eds.), *Suicide as a dramatic performance*. New Brunswick, NJ: Transaction.

Stack, S. (2015c). Suicide away from home. In D. Lester & S. Stack (Eds.), *Suicide as a dramatic performance*. New Brunswick, NJ: Transaction.

Steer, R. A., Beck, A. T., Garrison, B. & Lester, D. (1988). Eventual suicide in interrupted and uninterrupted attempters. *Suicide & Life-Threatening Behavior*, *18*, 119-128.

Triandis, H. (1993). Collectivism and individualism as cultural syndromes. *Cross-Cultural Research*, *27*, 155-180.

Williams, C. L., Davidson, J. A. & Montgomery, I. (1980). Impulsive suicidal behavior. *Journal of Clinical Psychology*, *36*, 90-94.

Wolfgang, M. E. (1958). *Patterns of criminal homicide*. Philadelphia, PA: University of Pennsylvania Press.

Yang, B. & Lester, D. (2011). The presentation of the self: an hypothesis about suicide notes. *Suicidology Online*, *2*, 75-79.

In: The End of Suicidology
Editor: David Lester
ISBN: 978-1-53615-310-1


*Chapter 8*

# AN ETHOLOGICAL APPROACH TO SUICIDE[1]

***David Lester, PhD***
Stockton University, Galloway, New Jersey, US

Ethology is the study of animal behavior, focusing on how and why animal behavior occurs.[2] Ethologists stress accurate observation and description of animal behavior, particularly in the animals' natural habitats, but also in experimental situations where the stimuli with which the animals are confronted can be presented in a systematic fashion. Ethology believes that the mechanisms behind animal behavior are programmed into the animal's neural networks and, thus, are determined largely by the genes and by the ways in which evolution has changed the characteristics of the animal.

It may not immediately be clear how ethological concepts could be applied to suicidal behavior, as some would argue that there must be evidence of conscious suicidal intent in order to classify a death as suicidal in nature (Goldstein, 1940). However, others, such as Menninger (1938), have disagreed with this narrow definition.

---

[1] This section was co-authored with Robert Goldney and based on Goldney and Lester (1997) and Lester and Goldney (1997).

[2] This presentation of the principles of ethology is based on Gould (1982) and Immelmann (1980).

Behavior which appears to be suicidal to an observer has been reported in dolphins (Amory, 1970), and biologists frequently use the term "suicide" to describe behavior in lower animals such as the pink bollworm moth (Bariola, 1978), butterflies (Trail, 1980), pea aphids (McAllister and Roitberg, 1987), birds (O'Connor, 1978) and bacteria such as motil aeromonads (Namdari and Cabelli, 1989). Therefore, there appears to be a sound basis for examining how an ethological approach could assist our understanding of suicidal behavior in humans.

This chapter reviews basic ethological principles briefly and then draws analogies with suicidal behavior.

## The Basic Concepts of Ethology

The basic concepts of ethology were developed by Konrad Lorenz and Niko Tinbergen who were awarded the Nobel Prize for Medicine for their work. Consider the following example, the egg-rolling response of the greylag goose. When a goose which is incubating eggs notices an egg near the nest, its attention is focused on this egg. The goose slowly rises, extends its neck over the egg and, with the bottom of its bill, rolls the egg back up into the nest. This behavior is called a *fixed action pattern*. The response appears to be innate rather than learned, the coordination and patterning of the behavior is stereotyped, and, once initiated, the pattern is completed without any further sensory input. The stimuli which release the fixed action pattern is called the *innate releasing mechanism*. Because the goose responds to only one aspect of the object, the stimuli are also called the *sign stimuli*. The fixed action pattern is turned off and on by *drives* or *motivation* which limits the behavior to a particular period of time, in this case incubation until hatching. Innate releasing mechanisms are thought to illustrate the innate, programmed nature of much of animal behavior. They focus the animal's attention and enable animals to respond quickly to stimuli without interference from thinking. These stimuli appear initially to be discrete rather than more complex patterns, but they can be modified over time so that the animal comes to substitute a rapidly acquired complex picture of the object for the innate releaser on which they depended initially.

Tinbergen experimented with the greylag goose's fixed action pattern and found that a variety of convex objects would trigger the egg rolling behavior in the goose. In fact, the goose preferred objects larger than eggs, preferring a volleyball over a goose egg, for example. The volleyball, in this instance, is a *supernormal stimulus*.

These behaviors are quite rigid. For example, the digger wasp catches crickets and returns them to its burrow, setting the cricket down about an inch from the burrow. The wasp then checks the burrow and returns for the cricket. If, while the wasp is checking the burrow, the cricket is moved by the experimenter further from the nest, the wasp moves it closer to the nest and then checks the burrow. If the experimenter keeps moving the cricket, the wasp never gets the cricket into the burrow.

Innate releasing mechanisms and fixed action patterns can be arranged in sequences so that one fixed action pattern involves stimuli which act as innate releasing mechanisms for the next fixed action pattern -- sequences most easily observed in the courtship patterns of animals. Another example of behavioral programming is *imprinting*, a behavior in which, for example, for a few hours after hatching, a bird responds to particular stimuli presented to it and follows the object presenting these stimuli. The bird accepts this object as a parent and, still later, will court this object.

The amplitude of the stimulus necessary to release the behavior is called its *threshold*. Performance of a behavior sometimes increases the threshold required for a repeat performance, for example, in copulation behavior, a phenomenon called *action-specific fatigue*. The animal can also habituate to the innate releasing mechanism and fail to respond to the stimulus, a phenomenon called *stimulus-specific fatigue*. This fatigue is presumed to occur at the neural level.

Each fixed action pattern has its own reaction-specific energy, similar to Freud's hydraulic model of energy (Cofer & Appley, 1964, p. 597). If the behavior pattern has not occurred for some time, then the fixed action pattern can be released by simpler and less specific stimuli. For example, dogs who do not get the opportunity to break the necks of prey, will attempt to this with slippers or other household objects, *substitute objects*. In extreme circumstances, the fixed action pattern may occur without any external stimuli present, *vacuum behavior*.

## Attempted Suicide as an Innate Releasing Mechanism

The first application of ethology to suicidal behavior was made by Stengel and Cook (1958). Referring to the work of Lorenz and Tinbergen, they suggested that "the suicidal attempt acts very much as a 'social releaser'" (p. 117). Stengel (1962) later wrote that "the suicidal attempt functions as an alarm system and an appeal for help. It does so almost with the regularity of an 'innate release mechanism'" (p. 726). It is of interest that these concepts are embodied in the title of Farberow and Shneidman's (1961) influential book, "The Cry for Help," where the suicide attempt, the innate releasing mechanism, is the stimulus which elicits a response, the fixed action pattern, in other people. The response elicited in others is evidently care-giving. This notion was also suggested by Henderson (1974) who characterized attempted suicide as care-eliciting behavior and saw it as a developmentally primitive signal for care.[3]

## Attempted Suicide as a Fixed Action Pattern

Attempted suicide can also be seen as a fixed action pattern. In Freud's early version of psychoanalytic theory, there was only one source of energy for human behavior, an energy which he called libido. In this version of the theory, the natural response to frustration is to aggress against the frustrating object, that is, to become assaultive. If this outward-directed aggression is forbidden or punished, then the aggression is blocked and turned inward

[3] For such appeals to work, they must elicit altruistic or care-giving behavior in the significant others, but the lack of such behavior does not negate the ethological analogy.

onto the self, resulting in depression and self-destructive behavior (Henry & Short, 1954).

However, in the later version of his theory, Freud proposed two major motivations for humans, the life and death instincts, Eros and Thanatos, fueled respectively by libido and destrudo. In this latter theory, adopted by Menninger (1938) in his theorizing about suicide, self-destructive behavior becomes a basic pattern which, in order to survive, we must control. In this view, suicidal behavior is an innate pattern of behavior, a fixed-action pattern in ethological terms.

If suicidal behavior can be viewed as a fixed action pattern, two questions arise. First, what is the innate releasing mechanism that elicits this behavior? At the most general level, stressors could be seen as the stimuli which elicit the behavior, but research has shown that the stressors which most commonly precipitate suicidal behavior vary with age, gender, and other personal characteristics (Lester, 1992).

More interestingly for an ethological perspective is the possibility that interpersonal stimuli are critical in eliciting suicidal behavior, a possibility most clearly illustrated in Richman's (1986) focus on the role of the family in both eliciting and reducing the occurrence of suicidal behavior. If this is the case, then we have sequencing, in which the behavior of one person releases the suicidal behavior pattern in another, which in turn releases care-giving behavior in the first person. More abstract analysis has been conducted on the dynamic interchange between the murderer and the victim (e.g., Luckenbill, 1977) than has been conducted on the back-and-forth communications between the suicidal individual and his or her significant others, and this gap needs to be addressed in future research on suicidal behavior.

The second question is, if suicidal behavior is a fixed action pattern, what will happen when no innate releasing mechanism appears? According to ethology, fixed action patterns must be expressed from time to time. As time passes without the occurrence of the fixed action pattern, the stimuli required to release the pattern become weaker and weaker, until the pattern can occur without any releasing stimulus, vacuum behavior.

## Discussion

In writing about outward-directed aggression, Lorenz (1966) addressed this problem by suggesting that socially acceptable outlets must be provided for the outward expression of aggression, outlets such as contact sports and paramilitary organizations. The same may, therefore, be true for suicidal behavior. The society must provide socially acceptable ways for self-destructive impulses to be safely discharged, for example, in death-risking activities such as mountain climbing or in chronic and focal suicidal activities, to use Menninger's (1938) terminology, such as drug use and self-mutilation. Just as the dog shakes a slipper rather than breaking the neck of its captured prey, perhaps people can abuse alcohol and other drugs rather than commit suicide with overdoses. From this perspective, therefore, drug abuse may be a means of preventing suicide!

## References

Amory, C. (1970). After living with a man, a dolphin may commit suicide. *Holiday*, May, 16-18.

Bariola, L. A. (1978). Suicidal emergence and reproduction by overwintered pink bollworm moths. *Environmental Entomology*, *7*, 189-192.

Cofer, C. N. & Appley, M. H. (1964). *Motivation*. New York: Wiley.

Farberow, N. L. & Shneidman, E. S. (Eds.) (1961). *The cry for help*. New York: McGraw-Hill.

Goldney, R. D. & Lester, D. (1997). Ethology and self-injury. *British Journal of Psychiatry*, *170*, 192-193.

Goldstein, K. (1940). *Human nature in the light of psychopathology*. Cambridge, MA: Harvard University.

Gould, J. L. (1982). *Ethology*. New York: Norton.

Henderson, S. (1974). Care-eliciting behavior in man. *Journal of Nervous and Mental Disease*, *159*, 172-181.

Henry, A. F. & Short, J. F. (1954). *Suicide and homicide*. New York: Free Press.

Immelmann, K. (1980). *Introduction to ethology*. New York: Plenum.

Lester, D. (1992). *Why people kill themselves*. Springfield, IL: Charles Thomas.

Lester, D. & Goldney, R. D. (1997). An ethological perspective on suicidal behavior. *New Ideas in Psychology*, *15*, 97-103.

Lorenz, K. (1966). *On aggression*. New York: Harcourt, Brace & World.

Luckenbill, D. (1977). Criminal homicide as a situated transaction., *Social Problems*, *25*, 176-186.

McAllister, M. K. & Roitberg, B. D. (1987). Adaptive suicidal behavior in pea aphids. *Nature*, *328*, 797-799.

Menninger, K. (1938). *Man against himself.* New York: Harcourt, Brace & World.

Namdari, H. & Cabelli, V. J. (1989). The suicide phenomenon in motile aeromonads. *Applied & Environmental Microbiology*, *55*, 543-547.

O'Connor, R. J. (1978). Brood reduction in birds. *Animal Behavior*, *26*, 79-96.

Richman, J. (1986). *Family therapy for suicidal people*. New York: Springer.

Stengel, E. (1962). Recent research into suicide and attempted suicide. *American Journal of Psychiatry*, *118*, 725-727.

Stengel, E. & Cook, N. G. (1958). *Attempted suicide: Its social significance and effects*, Maudsley Monograph Number 4. London, UK: Oxford University Press.

Trail, D. R. (1980). Behavioral interactions between parasites and hosts. *American Naturalist*, *116*(1), 77-91.

In: The End of Suicidology
Editor: David Lester
ISBN: 978-1-53615-310-1


*Chapter 9*

# EVOLUTION AND SUICIDE

***David Lester, PhD***
Stockton University, Galloway, New Jersey, US

There are several evolutionary ideas that are relevant to suicide. It has long been noticed that animal populations adjust to the size and abundance of nutrients in the environment. When resources are abundant, the population grows; when resources are scarce the population shrinks. Does the human animal fit this pattern? Many human practices can be viewed as serving to achieve population regulation. War, infanticide, geronticide, and murder in general can be seen as reducing the population in times of scarce resources. Social regulations on marriage, taboos on child spacing, and homosexuality can also be seen as ways of controlling population size.

Addressing the problem of drug addiction, Jonas and Jonas (1980) noted that, although addiction to drugs initially seems gratifying to the individual, the addict eventually suffers from declining health and a disrupted social adjustment. The fertility of the addict is impaired, and his genes are typically removed from the gene pool. (Natural selection involves the survival of the genes of individuals who are fit while those of less fit individuals are weeded out over time.)

Jonas and Jonas speculated that the genes of the addict (and perhaps the genes of those with psychiatric illnesses) predispose them to be sensitive to external stimuli and group pressures. These tendencies may have been adaptive when societies were smaller and when man had to be acutely sensitive to danger from the environment in order to survive. But in modern society, this sensitivity leads to discomfort which can sometimes be alleviated, for example, by the person blunting his perception by means of drugs.

Jonas and Jonas saw addicts today as forming an available pool of individuals readily amenable to a reduction in the population. (The large increase in stress diseases can also be seen as ways of reducing the population.) Jonas and Jonas noted that self-elimination behaviors have adaptive significance for the species. Addiction and similar behaviors are pathways along which some people move toward removing their genes from the gene pool.

## Application to Suicide

Suicidal behavior fits well into this process. Suicide clearly removes the genes of those individuals from the gene pool and reduces the size of the population. Furthermore, when we look at the kinds of individuals who complete suicide, we find that, typically, suicide rates are highest in those who are older and past child-bearing age, except in the poorest nations of the world where suicide rates are higher among the young and fertile female members of the society (15 to 24-year-olds) than among the older women (Lester, 1982). Thus, it seems that when resources are scarce, as in the poorest nations, it is the fertile who kill themselves at the highest rate, thereby reducing the potential for growth in the population. The fact that suicide rates are much higher in those who are psychiatrically disturbed (Lester, 1992) can also be seen as genetically useful, for the suicide of these people removes their (possibly defective) genes from the gene pool in the society. The existence of fatalistic and altruistic suicide (Durkheim, 1897), in which people kill themselves in conformity to societal pressures, may also be seen as fitting the type of suicide necessary for this evolutionary view better than the suicides of the isolates and the alienated of the society (egoistic and anomic suicides). The ritualistic suicides, for example, suttee in Indian widows and seppuku in Japan, are suicides committed in response to social pressures. Mass suicide can also be seen as satisfying this evolutionary need.

## DeCatanzaro: Sociobiology and Suicide

Sociobiology is a discipline which is an "amalgamation of behavioral biology, modern population ecology, and evolutionary theory…..Its central concern is to understand how and why animal social behavior has evolved" (Wittenberger, 1981, p. 6). Animal behavior orients the species toward maintaining and advancing its biological fitness, maintaining its existence and promoting its reproduction (DeCatanzaro, 1981).

DeCatanzaro (1981) noted that suicide appears to act contrary to this trend by removing the individual's genes from the population gene pool. However, DeCatanzaro noted that suicide occurs primarily in those who are under stress which reduces their biological fitness and who have a reduced capacity to promote their genes in future generations. Suicide has been more common in those who are older, who have no children, who are divorced, widowed and single, and in those who are psychiatrically disturbed, factors which reduce the capacity and ability to have children and pass on genes to future generations. However, since suicide is related to decreased reproductive status, it does not necessarily remove genes from the population gene pool, but the suicidal individual may, by dying by suicide, support related individuals in their quest for survival and reproduction, individuals who share some of their genes because they are members of the same family by descent. For example, the suicide of the elderly in primitive societies removes a burden on the remaining members of the society who no longer have to feed the aged and infirm and whose migration is no longer hindered by the weak elderly.

Perhaps this made sense in 1981 when DeCatanzaro wrote his book. However, the rising youth suicide rate in the 1980s and 1990s in most nations of the world seemed to argue against this point of view. The youths who died by suicide would in all probability have had children later had they not killed themselves. Furthermore, DeCatanzaro is very selective in his presentation of suicide statistics. For example, he notes that the high suicide rates in the widowed and divorced fits with his theory (since these individuals are presumably less likely to reproduce than married people), but he ignores phenomena such as the *reduced* suicide rate in women *after* they pass their period of child-bearing. Furthermore, the sociobiological perspective on suicidal behavior ignores nonfatal suicidal behavior. The sociobiological hypothesis about suicidal behavior thus seems to explain only some aspects of fatal suicidal behavior at some points in time and in some nations of the world.

## Suicide as a Derangement of the Self-Sacrificial Aspect of Eusociality

Joiner, et al. (2016) proposed a theory of suicide similar to that proposed by DeCatanzaro. *Eusociality* is a system of social organization in which there is cooperative care of the young members of the colony, and a form of labor in which members of the community defend the community, often sacrificing their own lives. Although rare (it has been documented in only roughly twenty species), aspects of it may be found in humans. In some bees, for example, the bee permanently locks its jaws onto an intruder, thereby killing the attacker and dying itself in the process.

In humans, one of the motivating forces for suicide is perceived burdensomeness (Joiner, 2005), in which the suicidal individual thinks that his family members (who have shared genes) and friends (community members) would be better off if he or she were dead. Joiner noted that research shows that at least 90% of suicides have a psychiatric disorder, and he proposed that the true rate may be 100% if psychiatrists were able to accurately diagnose each and every suicide. In these psychiatrically disturbed individuals, the choice of suicide because of perceived burdensomeness is a flawed and tragic miscalculation, labeled by Joiner, et al as a *derangement*. Thus, individuals who are deranged are unable to control the wired-in self-sacrificial aspect of eusociality.

## Suicidal Crises as Antipredator Defensive Reactions

It is, therefore, possible to view the roots of suicidal behavior as a result of our behaviors derived from evolutionary ancestors. Joiner and Stanley (2016) have proposed another way to do this. They noted that mammals display antipredator defensive reactions when threatened with possible attack and death. These reactions include a depression of activity and signaling other members of their species about the threat. When threatened with attack, some species freeze, while others prepare to attack or flee (fight versus flight).

Similar reactions occur in humans when threatened with attack, and Joiner and Stanley cited examples of such reactions in people who are threatened in mass murder situations. In the suicidal crisis, Joiner and Stanley noted that the suicidal individual is in two situations. He or she is threatened both with death and the killing (at their own hands). This may trigger the antipredator defense reactions which are pre-wired into our brains. Joiner and Stanley further noted that escape is impossible since the killer (himself or herself) is close at hand and inescapable.

The two major reactions in humans in crisis (including suicidal crises) are over-arousal (agitation, insomnia, nightmares, irritability, rage, etc.) and shutdown phenomena (social withdrawal, cessation of activities, anorexia, mutism, etc.). These reactions parallel the freezing versus flight and fight reactions in animals. Relevant to this is the finding by De Leo (2010), in his interviews with serious suicide attempters, of acute anxiety and over-arousal in them immediately prior to their suicide attempts.

## SOPER'S EVOLUTIONARY THEORY

Cas Soper (2014, 2016) asked why psychiatric disorders are so common. Soper noted that major depressive disorders occur in 7% of the American population and addictive disorders in 47%. From the perceptive of evolutionary psychology, this high frequency of psychiatric disorders must have its origin in natural selection. Psychiatric disorders must provide a reproductive advantage that compensates for the disabling impact of these disorders.

Soper noted that explanations have been proposed for specific psychiatric disorders. For example, depression may stop people wasting resources on futile projects, a way to avoid attack from a stronger rival, or a method social of manipulation. Soper noted, however, that such specific explanations fail to address the issue that comorbidity, in which a person has two or more psychiatric disorders concurrently, is so common. Soper argued that any explanation for depression must also account for depression commonly being comorbid with addiction. Soper also noted that psychiatric disorders often "churn over time," that is, people have different disorders at different points in time.

Soper noted that suicide is more common in those with a psychiatric disorder, from which it is typically concluded that psychiatric disorder causes suicide. Soper cites Martin (1997, p. 304) as saying that "Depression drives thousands of people to kill themselves each year." Soper proposed instead that suicide triggers psychiatric disorder or that the common mental illnesses are adaptations designed to *counter* the possibility of suicide. Psychiatric disorders developed, therefore, as a defence against self-destruction.

To support this hypothesis, Soper noted that addicts often refer to their use of alcohol and drugs as a solution to their problem, that is, they are self-medicating. Thus, addiction may act to prevent individuals from taking their own lives. Similarly, depression may serve to incapacitate people and lessen the risk of acting on suicidal impulses. Similarly, non-fatal acts of self-harm may lessen the risk of fatal suicidal behavior.

Soper also addressed the issue of why have humans evolved a capacity for suicide. Soper suggested that suicide arises from a lack of meaning in people's lives and that this is an unfortunate side-effect of (or trade-off for) the advantage of self-awareness or self-consciousness.

In his more recent book (Soper, 2018), Soper has enlarged his evolutionary theory of suicide. Suicide is motivated by pain for which the brain seeks escape, an idea consistent with Baumeister's (1990) escape theory of suicide and the defeat-entrapment theory of suicide (see Gunn, 2014). There are cultural defenses against the idea of suicide, including making suicide a taboo behavior and stigmatizing it, and introducing the idea of an after-life which has punishments for suicide. There are also mechanisms for dealing with chronic pain, including autonomic numbing, compulsive self-medication, detachment from unbearable and painful reality, degrading the ability to plan and enact tasks, and loss of psychomotor energy. Several of these tactics involve behaviors that are symptomatic of psychiatric disorder.

## COMMENT

The theorists in the present chapter have suggested ways in which suicidal behavior may be understand from an evolutionary perspective, complementing the ideas presented above in Chapter 8. The critical question is whether these evolutionary theories can generate hypotheses which are inconsistent with other theories and, also, stimulate research.

## REFERENCES

Baumeister, R. F. (1990). Suicide as escape from self. *Psychological Review*, *97*, 90-113.

DeCatanzaro, D. (1981). *Suicide and self-damaging behavior*. New York: Academic.

De Leo, D. (2010). *Turning points*. Bowen Hills, Australia: Australian Academic Press.

Durkheim, E. (1897). *Le Suicide* [*Suicide*]. Paris: Felix Alcan.

Gunn, J. F. (2014). The role of defeat and entrapment in suicidal behavior. In J. F. Gunn & D. Lester. *Theories of suicide*, pp. 37-54. Springfield, IL: Charles Thomas.

Joiner, T. E. (2005). *Why people die by suicide*. Cambridge, MA: Harvard University Press.

Joiner, T. E., Hom, M. A., Hagan, C. R. & Silva, C. (2016). Suicide as a derangement of the self-sacrificial aspect of eusociality. *Psychological Review*, *123*, 235-254.

Joiner, T. E. & Stanley, I. H. (2016). Can the phenomenology of a suicidal crisis be usefully understood as a suite of antipredator defensive reactions? *Psychiatry*, *79*, 107-109.

Jonas, D. & Jonas, A. (1980). A bioanthropological overview of addiction. In D. Lettieri, M. Sayers, & H. Pearson (Eds.) *Theories on drug abuse*, pp. 269-277. Rockville: NIDA.

Lester, D. (1982). The distribution of sex and age among completed suicides: a cross-national study. *International Journal of Social Psychiatry*, *28*, 256-260.

Lester, D. (1992). *Why people kill themselves*. Springfield, IL: Charles Thomas.

Martin, P. (1997). *The sickening mind*. London, UK: Harper Collins.

Soper, C. (September 2014). *Anti-suicide mechanisms as a general evolutionary explanation for common mental disorders*. Unpublished working paper, University of Gloucestershire. Available on researchgate.net.

Soper, C. (May 30, 2016). *Could some common mental diseases be evolved defences against suicide?* Unpublished working paper, University of Gloucestershire. Available on researchgate.net.

Soper, C. (2018). *The evolution of suicide*. New York: Springer.

Wittenberger, J. F. (1981). *Animal social behavior*. Boston: Duxbury.

In: The End of Suicidology
Editor: David Lester
ISBN: 978-1-53615-310-1


*Chapter 10*

# SUICIDE, CHAOS THEORY, NON-LINEARITY, AND THE TIPPING POINT[1]

***David Lester, PhD***
Stockton University, Galloway, New Jersey, US

Two analogies can be drawn from the natural sciences which may be applicable to suicidology and provide important insights. The first concerns the differences in predicting the behavior of the individual versus the aggregate.

## THE INDIVIDUAL VERSUS THE AGGREGATE

Radioactive atoms are unstable and decay into other atoms. The speed of decay is measured by the half-life, that is, the time period required for half of the atoms in a sample of the element to decay into the new elements. Half-lives of the atoms of different elements can vary from less than one second to over a billion years. For example, after 29 years, half of the atoms

[1] This chapter is based on Lester (1994).

of strontium-90 will have decayed into yttrium-90. After another 29 years, one half of the remaining atoms will have decayed, and so on (Shapiro, 1979). Physicists cannot predict which particular atoms will decay during the half-life, or when any particular atom will decay. Those atoms which decay during the half-life look, initially, identical to those which do not decay.

The analogy with suicide is strong. While it is impossible to predict which people will die by suicide next year, we do know that, in America for example, some 45,000 will do so. Predicting the behavior of the aggregate is possible, while predicting the behavior of the individual is very difficult.

Actually, the task for the suicidologist is a little easier than that confronting the physicist, for the potential suicides do differ from the potential non-suicides at the beginning of the observation period. Various risk factors have been identified for suicide, such as gender, the presence of an affective disorder, current substance abuse, and a history of physical and sexual abuse. Despite this, any attempt to predict which individuals will die by suicide in the next year leads to an enormous number of false positives. Furthermore, Franklin, et al. (2017) reviewed 365 research studies from the past 50 years in order to identify risk factors for suicidal thoughts and behaviors. They found that prediction was only slightly better than chance for all outcomes (ideation, attempts and death) and that predictive ability had not improved over the last 50 years.

## Input-Output: What Makes Someone Die by Suicide?

A second analogy is that it may be surprising to find out that, in many problems, small differences in input can produce large differences in output (Gleick, 1987). In meteorology, Lorenz (1979, 1984) attempted to model climate using a simplified mathematical model. The traditional view was that later conditions could be predicted from an approximate knowledge of initial conditions with reasonably accuracy. Small influences will *not* have large effects eventually. On one occasion, Lorenz tried to replicate the second half of a sequence of his artificial climate by entering the values obtained in the middle of a previous run. He found that the slight initial discrepancies grew larger and larger, until the new sequence was completely unlike the original sequence. He had entered decimals rounded to three places rather than six. This small change proved to be catastrophic.[2]

The interesting feature of weather prediction is that we can predict the obvious, for example, that next July will be sunnier and hotter than January (the periodic component), but this is uninteresting. What people want to predict is whether a particular day will have rain. It is the non-periodic component that we want to predict. When and where will a tornado hit? When will the rain be so heavy that the river will flood?

In the prediction of human behavior, suicidologists can predict the regularities. For example, using Erikson's (1959) stages of human development, we can predict the normal course of development. However, that is not very interesting. We want to be able to predict the particular course of development for a particular individual. For suicidal behavior which is statistically rare and non-periodic we want to predict whether and when this individual will die by suicide, not what the suicide rate of the population will be next year.

What may make this difficult is not necessarily the complexity of the information we have to obtain about individuals throughout their lives in order to make the prediction, but that this catastrophic event, suicide, may be produced, not by some *major* event or events occurring at some prior point in time, but rather by some minor differences in an otherwise ordinary life course.

Lorenz speculated on the possibility that a butterfly stirring its wings in Brazil today may produce a tornado in Texas next month. Perhaps slightly too much or too little of some ordinary parental behavior may lead to suicide for their child later in life? In suicidology, we expect, and therefore search for, major events which might lead to suicide in the future, whereas perhaps the causes of suicide are subtle.

---

[2] Chaos theory is a branch of mathematics focused on the behavior of dynamical systems that are highly sensitive to initial conditions.

In the *cusp catastrophe model*, a system has two states, and the system can shift from one state to the other suddenly with only a minor input. The result is that this shift appears to be (and may, in fact, be) unpredictable. If we apply this to the suicidal individual, it may be possible for some people to switch from a non-suicidal state to a suicidal state with only a minor input or provocation and, as a consequence, we tend to view the suicidal person as impulsive. However, the suicidal state (as well as the non-suicidal state) may be long-standing, and the suicidal state may have taken over the consciousness of the individual on many occasions in the past.

## NON-LINEAR MODELS

A number of recent authors have suggested a non-linear approach to the study of suicidal behavior: Mishara (1996), Ramsay (1997), Rogers (2003), Large (2010), Rogers and Lester (2010), Schiepek, et al., (2011), and Sawhney (2012). Fartacek, et al. (2016) defined a non-linear approach as dynamic (evolving over time) and where the input and output are not proportional to each other. For example, marginal stressors (input) may trigger suicide (output), while severe stressors (input) may not trigger suicide (output). The failure to predict, and even understanding, suicide does not reflect that we are unaware of critical risk factors or have inadequate theories of suicide, but rather that there is inherent complexity in the suicidal process.

Sheehan and Giddens (2015) criticized the staircase step model of suicidal behavior. For example, if an individual has a suicidal plan, this assumes that there is prior suicidal intent, and the existence of a plan assumes great importance in the sequence. The implication is that each suicidal individual progresses in an orderly way toward dying by suicide – from passive suicidal ideation, to active suicidal ideation, to suicidal intent, making a suicidal plan, and attempting suicide to dying by suicide. In this ladder, when the individual is at one step, it is assumed that he or she has passed through all the previous steps in order. Sheehan and Giddens noted that some individuals may proceed through these steps in a linear fashion, but not all do, and maybe not even the majority do so.

Many suicidal individuals, on any given day, may experience any one of these elements of suicidality in a non-linear time-sequence and in many possible combinations. They may experience active suicidal ideation, followed by passive suicidal ideation, begin to write a suicide note, and then experience the dissipation of suicidality for the rest of the day. As Sheehan and Giddens describe this process"

> Suicidality is non-linear, as experienced by a suicidal individual over time. It is dynamic, involving a complex interaction of core suicidal experiences ("phenomena") over time....It is not linear, not unidimensional, not necessarily cumulative, and not necessarily like a staircase. (p. 24)

Fartacek, et al. (2016) gave one person daily psychological tests for a period of 91 days prior to her suicide attempt. The charts for the daily self-reported measures of pressure, perturbation, hope, suicide risk, wish to die and wish to live were very irregular, with no simple trends over the 91 days. Her daily report of suicide risk was high at the beginning of the period and in the middle and highest in the days at the end of the period, but from days 75 to 85, she rated her risk of suicide as zero, her wish to live as high and her wish to die as low.

## THE TIPPING POINT

The tipping point refers to any process in which, beyond a certain point, the rate of the process increases dramatically (Gladwell, 2000). In sociology, a tipping point is a point in time when a group, or a large number of group members, rapidly and dramatically changes its behavior by widely adopting a previously rare practice. For example, Grodzins (1957), in his study of American neighborhoods, found that, as long as the number of African-American families moving in remained small, then white families stayed put. But when "one too many" African-American families moved in, then white families moved out *en masse*. Grozdins called this the *tipping point*.

Tipping points are of interest because the event that causes the change may not be large. Imagine a pile of coal (or sand or some other object). As you add more and more coal to the pile, it may remain stable for a while, but then one extra piece of coal causes a collapse of the pile. Or consider water piling up behind a dam. The dam holds until one extra, perhaps small, rainfall causes the dam to burst. Goldney (1998) raised the possibility of the presence of a tipping point in the rise in the suicide rate of young males in many countries. Goldney suggested that a minor change in a social factor might have suddenly breached the tipping point for suicide, and he saw this idea as congruent with Mishara's dynamic model of suicide (see Chapter 5). Goldney noted that this idea also suggests that suicide prevention might more usefully focus on changing social variables at the community or national level in order to move the number of suicides away from the tipping point, rather than focusing on the small number of high risk individuals. For example, the switch from coal gas to natural gas for domestic use (which was not done to prevent suicide, but rather for economic reasons) had a tremendous impact on the suicide rates in the countries that changed the type of domestic gas. The number of suicides in those countries dropped dramatically, thereby moving the numbers away from the possible tipping point.

When we analyze a particular suicide, we typically look for some major stressful event to have occurred that would have made the suicide understandable. Tipping point theory suggests, in contrast, that the event may have been relatively minor, like that extra bit of rain that burst the dam.

## Comment

The ideas in this chapter have portrayed suicide as more complex than we might, at first, think. Input-output models, cusp-catastrophe models, non-linear models and tipping points indicate that our theoretical models for suicide may have to be more complex than the simple models typically proposed by psychologists, sociologists and psychiatrists for suicide and other behaviors.

## References

Erikson, E. (1959). *Identity and life cycle*. New York: International University Press.

Fartacek, C., Schiepek, G., Kunrath, S., Fartacek, R. & Plöderl, M. (2016). Real-time monitoring of non-linear suicidal dynamics. *Frontiers in Psychology*, *7*, #130, 1- 14.

Franklin, J. C., Ribeiro, J. D., Fox, K. R., Bentley, K. H., Kleinman, E. M., Huang, X. & Nock, M. K. (2017). Risk factors for suicidal thoughts and behaviors. *Psychological Bulletin*, *143*, 187-232.

Gladwell, M. (2000). *The tipping point*. Boston, MA: Little Brown.

Gleick, J. (1987). *Chaos*. New York: Viking.

Goldney, R. (1998). Variation in suicide rates: The tipping point. *Crisis*, *19*, 136-137.

Grozdins, M. M. (1957) Metropolitan segregation. *Scientific American*, *197*, (4, October), 33-41.

Large, M. (2010). No evidence for improvement in the accuracy of suicide risk assessment. *Journal of Nervous & Mental Disease*, *198*, 604.

Lester, D. (1994). Reflections on the statistical rarity of suicide. *Crisis*, *15*, 187-188.

Lorenz, E. (1979). Predictability: does the flap of a butterfly wings in Brazil set off a tornado in Texas? Paper presented at the *American Association for the Advancement of Science*. Washington, DC.

Lorenz, E. (1984). Irregularity. *Tellus*, *36A*, 98-100.

Mishara, B. L. (1996). A dynamic developmental model of suicide. *Human Development*, *39*, 181-194.

Ramsay, R. (1997). Chaos theory and crisis intervention. *Child & Family*, *1*, 23-25.

Rogers, J. R. (2003). The anatomy of suicidology. *Suicide & Life-Threatening Behavior*, *33*, 9-20.

Rogers, J. R. & Lester, D. (2010). *Understanding suicide: why we don't and how we might.* Göttingen, Germany: Hogrefe.

Sawhney, V. (2012). Chaos theory and suicide. *Australasian Psychiatry*, *20*, 533.

Schiepek, G., Fartacek, C., Sturm, J., Kralovec, K. Fartacek, R. & Plöderl, M. (2011). Nonlinear dynamics. *Suicide & Life-Threatening Behavior*, *41*, 661-675.

Shapiro, G. (1979). *Physics without math*. Englewood Cliffs, NJ: Prentice Hall.

Sheehan, D. V. & Giddens, J. M. (2015). *Suicidality: a roadmap for assessment and treatment*. Tampa, FL: Harm Research Press.

In: The End of Suicidology
Editor: David Lester
ISBN: 978-1-53615-310-1


*Chapter 11*

# IS THERE A NATURAL SUICIDE RATE?

***Bijou Yang, PhD****
Economics and International Business,
Drexel University, Philadelphia, Pennsylvania, US

In times of full employment, the unemployment rate is unlikely to be zero. Even in times of full employment, some employees will quit or be fired and, between jobs, these individuals will be unemployed. This is called *frictional unemployment*, consisting of *search unemployment* and *wait unemployment*, that is, those searching for employment or waiting for employment. In addition, there is *structural unemployment* which results from changes over time in consumer demand and industrial development, and which affects the demand for labor both occupationally and geographically. Moreover, there is unemployment caused by seasonal demand such as construction work and agricultural migrant work. These three types of unemployment, present during times of full employment, constitute what has been called the *natural rate of unemployment* (e.g., McEachern, 2003). The implication is that there can never be a zero

* Emerita Professor.

unemployment rate. The best that can be attained is the natural rate of unemployment.

Lester and Yang (1997) (analyzed three theories relating the suicide rate to economic cycles and found that all of those theories predicted that the curve had a positive intercept on the y-axis during normal economic conditions. Durkheim's (1897) classic theory of suicide proposed that suicide rates would be higher at very high levels of social integration (the degree to which the members of a society are bound together in social networks) leading to *altruistic suicide* and at very low levels of social integration, leading to *egoistic suicide*. Durkheim's theory also predicted that suicide rates would be higher at very high levels of social regulation (the degree to which the members of the society have their desires controlled by societal norms and values), leading to *fatalistic suicide*, and at very low levels of social regulation, leading to *anomic suicide*. Durkheim did not stipulate that the suicide rate would be zero at intermediate levels of social integration and social regulation. Maris (1981), a sociologist, speculated that the suicide rate could never be zero no matter how ideal the social-economic conditions were. Yang and Lester (1991) proposed, therefore, that the suicide rate of a society could never be zero even if both the economic and the social conditions were made ideal from the point of view of suicide.[1]

Viren (1999) discussed whether there was a natural rate of suicide (or as he sometimes referred to it in his paper, a natural level of suicide). However, he changed the meaning of this term considerably. Viren acknowledged that the societal suicide rate was determined by both social factors and economic factors, and he proposed that the natural rate of suicide was the suicide rate that prevails when income is growing at the expected rate of long-term growth (Viren, 1999, p. 1429). This leaves the suicide rate as determined solely by social (or structural) factors. This is quite different from the definition suggested by Yang and Lester.

Viren presented data from a time-series analysis of the Finnish suicide rate from 1878-1994 to support his hypothesis that, once economic conditions were factored out, the suicide rate would be non-zero and

---

[1] Lester (1994) extended this and proposed the existence of a natural homicide rate.

positive. He examined the impact of GDP per capita, bankruptcies, unemployment and the stock price index, as well as controls for the sex distribution, average age of the population and urbanization. He found that economic variables were associated with the Finnish suicide rate. However, this data analysis does not appear to be pertinent to the issue of whether the suicide rate of a society can ever be zero.

## EMPIRICAL TESTS OF THE PROPOSAL OF A NATURAL SUICIDE RATE

Yang and Lester carried out a series of studies to explore whether there is a natural suicide rate for societies. Yang and Lester (1991) examined the 48 continental and contiguous states of the United States in 1980. Three variables were strongly and positively associated with the suicide rates of the states: the divorce rate, inter-state migration and church non-attendance. The multiple R in a full regression was 0.85. When the values of these three variables were set to zero in the regression equation, the suicide rate was determined solely by the constant term of 6.01. This means that, if no one was divorced in the USA, if there was no inter-state migration and if everyone went to church, the suicide rate would be 6.01 per 100,000 per year. Yang and Lester calculated this natural rate of suicide for men and women separately and found rates of 11.6 and 0.9, respectively.

Yang and Lester (2004) next studied ten nations for which data were available for the suicide rates of the regions of each nation (state, province or county). Data for the divorce and unemployment rates were available for each region of each nation and regression equations were calculated for each nation to predict the suicide rate. For example, the regression equation for Norway in 1980 was:

$$\text{Suicide rate} = 5.834 + 4.37 * \text{divorce rate} + 0.40 * \text{unemployment rate}$$

Setting the divorce and unemployment rates to zero gives an estimate of the natural suicide rate for Norway as 5.8 per 100,000 per year.

Yang and Lester presented the actual suicide rate and the estimated natural suicide rate for the ten nations as follows:

| Nation | Natural suicide rate | Actual suicide rate |
|---|---|---|
| Austria | 15.7 | 26.0 |
| Finland | 11.2 | 24.7 |
| France | 16.8 | 19.2 |
| Germany | 15.5 | 21.4 |
| Japan | 17.0 | 17.5 |
| Norway | 5.8 | 12.4 |
| Poland | 4.6 | 12.7 |
| Switzerland | 14.2 | 24.7 |
| Taiwan | 7.9 | 9.9 |
| USA | 8.1 | 12.0 |

The estimated natural suicide rate was in each case positive and less than the actual suicide rate. The Spearman rank correlation coefficient between the two rates was 0.57 and statistically significant. Yang and Lester concluded that the natural suicide rate may differ by nation. Why might this be so? Yang and Lester noted that nations do differ in variables that might affect the suicide rate. For example, it has been proposed that the Finno-Ugrian gene (found primarily in Finnish and Hungarian people) increases the risk of suicide (Voracek, et al., 2003), that the distribution of blood types is associated with psychiatric disorder and suicide (Lester, 2004), and that nations differ in the levels of various neurotransmitters in the brains, thereby possibly affecting the suicide rates (Lester, 1991). These physiologically-based factors may be important in determining the different natural suicide rates in different nations. However, these explanations are speculative at the present time and require further research.

Yang and Lester (2009) then extended their ecological (regional study) to include Russia, for which the estimated natural suicide rate was 24.6, and they corrected the previous values obtained for Poland (now 5.0) and the United States (now 8.2). Yang and Lester also examined the estimated natural suicide rate using time-series analyses for thirteen nations, again using divorce and unemployment rates to estimate the natural suicidal rate (and using both OLS regression and the Cochrane-Orcutt correction for serial autocorrelation). Their results were as follows:

| Nation | Estimated suicide rate (OLS) | Estimated suicide rate (corrected) |
|---|---|---|
| Australia | 12.5 | 12.6 |
| Austria | 15.9 | 15.7 |
| Belgium | 10.3 | 10.7 |
| Canada | 7.0 | 7.8 |
| Denmark | 11.2 | 11.6 |
| England/Wales | 11.5 | 10.5 |
| Japan | 25.0 | 7.3 |
| The Netherlands | 5.0 | 5.2 |
| Norway | 2.9 | 3.0 |
| Sweden | 19.3 | 20.4 |
| Taiwan | 10.3 | 9.9 |
| USA | 8.8 | 8.6 |
| West Germany | 18.0 | 20.6 |

Yang and Lester (2009) pointed out that there are many possible regression equations that can be derived in order to predict suicide rates (and from which estimates of the natural suicide rate can be made), both in ecological (regional) studies and in time-series studies. There may well be some regression equations for which the constant term (which is the estimate of the natural suicide rate) may be zero or negative, indicating that the natural suicide rate is zero, but they had not identified such situations in their research.

Empirical study of this issue is limited by two factors. First, data need to be available for regions of a nation or over time for variables that are associated with the suicide rate. Second, the variables chosen must be such that it is obvious what their value should be in an "ideal" society, that is, variables that minimize the suicide rate. It is obvious that, since unemployment is associated with an increase in the suicide rate (Platt, 1984), an ideal society would have a zero unemployment rate. It is not clear what the marriage rate, the birth rate or the emigration rate should be for a society to have a minimal suicide rate.

## OTHER EMPIRICAL TESTS OF THE NATURAL SUICIDE RATE HYPOTHESIS

Kunce and Anderson (2001-2002) used panel data from all 50 states of the United States plus the District of Columbia for the period 1985-1995. They also used age-adjusted rates which control for the fact that the state populations vary in their age distribution. Kunce and Anderson used eight variables to predict the suicide rate: unemployment rate, medical household income, divorce rate, residing in non-metropolitan areas, Christian church adherent, poverty rate, single occupancy households, and percent of the population that was non-white. The constant term was 1.28, and so Kunce and Anderson concluded that the natural suicide rate of the United States was 1.28.

This is, of course incorrect. Using their variables, the estimate of the American natural suicide rate is 1.28 only if all the eight variables are set to zero. This would mean, for example, zero Christian church adherents, and zero median household income, situations that would not be expected to result in zero suicides. The Christian church adherent variable should probably be set to one hundred percent, but it is by no means clear to what the median household income should be set. This is why Yang and Lester restricted their predictor variables to divorce and unemployment rates since it is clear that these should be set to zero in an ideal society.

Andrés and Halicioglu (2011) tested Yang and Lester's hypothesis of a natural suicide rate using data from 15 OECD nations for the period 1970-2004, using divorce and unemployment rates as the predictor variables.

Andrés and Halicioglu noted that Yang and Lester did not address the issue of spurious regression, carry out any diagnostic checks of their regression equations, explore the impact of lag in the response of suicide rate to socio-economic variables, and explore gender disparities. Andrés and Halicioglu remedied these omissions and found that, for the total suicide rate, the constant term was positive for 14 of the 15 nations (Finland was the exception) and statistically significant for 12 of the 14 nations. The constant term was positive for the male suicide rate in 14 of the 15 nations (again Finland was the exception) and positive for the female suicide rate for 14 of the 15 nations (the UK was the exception). The positive constant term was statistically significant for 12 of the 14 nations for the male suicide rate and for 12 of the 14 nations for the female suicide rate. Andrés and Halicioglu concluded that "[t]he results at the aggregate level confirm the study of Yang and Lester (1991) but our results are more robust" (p. 26).

Andrés and Halicioglu concluded that Turkey had the lowest natural suicide rate (3.64) and Japan the highest (13.98). For males the range was from the UK (4.73) to Belgium (15.44) while for females the range was from Italy (5.60) to Japan (16.76).

## Applications of the Natural Suicide Rate Hypothesis

Gmel, et al. (1998) investigated the association over time of alcohol consumption and suicide in Switzerland from 1950 to 1990. They found only a weak association and only for women. In looking at their data, Gmel et al. noticed a single harmonic long-term wave, peaking in 1950 and 1980 with a trough in 1965. They noted that harmonic trends are often seen as reflecting "natural" waves of phenomena, and they saw this as consistent with Yang and Lester's proposal of a natural rate of suicide. Harmonic waves reflect long-term fluctuations around a mean. Gmel et al. point out that, if this explanation is correct, then an explanation must be found for the harmonic wave.

## DISCUSSION

Goldney (2003) has proposed a similar idea to the natural suicide rate by hypothesizing that "there is a base rate of suicide in all communities" (Goldney, 2003, p. 141). Goldney suggested that, even in a theoretically ideal world with an optimum psychosocial environment, there would be a base rate of suicide in the range of 5 to 10 per 100,000 per year. Variations from this base rate are primarily a result of psychosocial factors. Rates lower than the base rate lack credibility and are a result of inadequate documentation. Typically, more accurate documentation of suicides results in a higher suicide rate, a phenomenon seen in Ireland where the influence of the Roman Catholic religion (which views suicide as a sin) resulted in suicides being classified as accidental or undetermined death (Cantor, et al., 1997) Rates higher than the base rate are a result of suicidogenic psychosocial factors such as easy access to lethal methods for suicide and poor socio-economic conditions (e.g., high divorce rates and high unemployment rates).

Goldney implied in his presentation of this hypothesis that the base rate of suicide is primarily a result of a "basic biological substrate (p. 145), that is, genetic and physiological factors.[2] He suggested, therefore, that a nation with a suicide rate close to the base rate should base their suicide prevention efforts on a traditional illness model, focusing on the management of psychiatric disorders and the appropriate use of psychiatric medications. Nations with a suicide rate higher than the base rate should focus instead on changing the psychosocial environment to lower the suicide rate, using tactics such as restricting access to lethal methods for suicide, proposing media guidelines for reporting suicides, and improving the socio-economic conditions that are risk factors for suicide.

[2] Kondrichin and Lester (1997) found that the percentage of Finno-Ugrians in European countries was associated with national suicide rates, while Lester (1991) found that the density of imipramine-binding sites in the brains of samples from countries was also associated with national suicide rates. These findings support Goldney's hypothesis.

## REFERENCES

Andrés, A. R. & Halicioglu, F. (2011). Testing the hypothesis of the natural suicide rates: further evidence from OECD data. *Economic Modelling, 28*, 22-26.

Cantor, C. H., Leenaars, A. A. & Lester, D. (1997). Under-reporting of suicide in Ireland 1960-1989. *Archives of Suicide Research*, *3*, 5-12.

Durkheim, E. (1897). *Le suicide* [*Suicide*]. Paris: Felix Alcan.

Gmel G., Rehm, J. & Ghazinouri, A. (1998). Alcohol and suicide in Switzerland. *Drug & Alcohol Review*, *17*, 27-37.

Goldney, R. D. (2003). A novel integrated knowledge explanation of factors leading to suicide. *New Ideas in Psychology*, *21*, 141-146.

Kondrichin, S. & Lester, D. (1997). Finno-Ugrians and suicide. *Perceptual & Motor Skills*, *85*, 514.

Kunce, M. & Anderson, A. L. (2001-2002). A natural rate of suicide for the U.S. revisited. *Omega*, *44*, 215-222.

Lester, D. (1991). The association between platelet imipramine bonding and suicide. *Pharmacopsychiatry*, *24*, 232.

Lester, D. (1994). Is there a natural homicide rate? *Psychological Reports*, *75*, 1434.

Lester, D. (1997). The association between platelet imipramine binding sites and suicide. *Pharmacopsychiatry*, *24*, 232.

Lester, D. (2004). Blood types and national suicide rates. *Crisis*, *25*, 140.

Lester, D. & Yang, B. (1997). *The economy and suicide*. Hauppauge, NY, US: Nova Science Publishers.

Maris, R. W. (1981). *Pathways to suicide.* Baltimore: Johns Hopkins University Press.

McEachern, W. A. (2003). *Macroeconomics.* Mason, OH: South-Western.

Platt, S. D. (1984). Unemployment and suicidal behavior. *Social Science & Medicine*, *19*, 93-115.

Viren, M. (1999). Testing the 'natural rate of suicide' hypothesis. *International Journal of Social Economics*, *26*, 1428-1440.

Voracek, M., Fisher, M. L. & Marusic, A. (2003). The Finno-Ugrian suicide hypothesis. *Perceptual & Motor Skills*, *97*, 401-406.

Yang, B. & Lester, D. (1991). Is there a natural suicide rate for a society? *Psychological Reports*, *68*, 322.

Yang, B. & Lester, D. (2004). Natural suicide rates in nations of the world. *Crisis*, *25*, 187-188.

Yang, B. & Lester, D. (2009). Is there a natural suicide rate? *Applied Economics Letters*, *16*, 137-140.

In: The End of Suicidology
Editor: David Lester
ISBN: 978-1-53615-310-1


*Chapter 12*

# SUICIDE AS A RANDOM WALK

***Bijou Yang, PhD****

Economics and International Business,
Drexel University, Philadelphia, Pennsylvania, US

Ever since Durkheim's (1897) seminal work on suicide was published, numerous theoretical and empirical works have been published in the field of suicidology in order to unveil the mystery of the societal suicide rate (e.g., Lester, 1989; Lester & Yang, 1997).[1] However, none of these investigations have looked into the variation of the suicide rate over time itself.[2] This chapter uses econometric techniques in order to explore the characteristics of the time-series suicide rate and to show that the findings are compatible with Durkheim's original data and theoretical framework.

---

* Emerita Professor.

[1] While Lester (1989) provides a detailed review of the theoretical literature, Lester and Yang (1997) focus more on empirical studies, especially about the relationship between the macroeconomic environment and the suicide rate. Both books review numerous investigations in the field of suicidology.

[2] The one exception might be the circadian variation in suicide attempts examined by Motohashi (1990).

## A Random Walk Hypothesis of the Suicide Rate

If we assume that the suicide rate is a stochastic process[3], then the time-series suicide rate could be stationary or nonstationary. Stationarity means that the characteristics of the stochastic process do not change over time, whereas nonstationarity means that those characteristics change over time.[4]

Among the nonstationary stochastic processes, the types of nonstationarity might be a result of the underlying stochastic process (difference nonstationarity) or to a linear trend (trend nonstationarity) (Nelson & Plosser, 1982). A good example of the former type of nonstationarity is the movement of stock prices over time, while a good example of the latter type of nonstationarity is a sinusoidal wave along an upward linear trend. The difference between these two types of nonstationary stochastic processes is that the former has a unit root. Any nonstationary stochastic process, if found to have a unit root, is called a random walk. Therefore, a random walk refers to a nonstationary stochastic process with a unit root.[5]

By drawing from research in econometrics, two relevant characteristics of a random walk can be identified: (1) the basic characteristics of a time-series are found to change over time, and (2) a portion of any disturbance to the stochastic process of concern will persist through time (Diebold & Nerlove, 1990, p. 37; Rudebusch, 1990).[6] The first property is derived from the fact that a random walk is nonstationary. The second property has

[3] A stochastic process is a time sequence representing the evolution of some system represented by a variable whose change is subject to a random variation.

[4] Most applications of the time-series analyses focus on the nonstationary process, especially in economics. For example, Nelson and Plosser (1982) found that most macroeconomic time-series are better characterized as nonstationary stochastic processes rather than as stationary fluctuations around a deterministic trend. Nonstationary stochastic processes have been applied also to financial market variables such as futures contracts (Samuelson, 1965), stock prices (Samuelson, 1973), dividends (Kleidon, 1986), and spot and forward exchange rates (Meese & Singleton, 1983).

[5] A unit root is a stochastic trend in a time series, sometimes called a "random walk with drift." If a time series has a unit root, it shows a systematic pattern that is unpredictable.

[6] One property of a random walk included in Yang's (1992) paper indicated that individuals use available information rationally. Applied to suicide, this brings up a psychological issue which was, apparently, ignored by Durkheim (1897) since he was concerned only with sociological dimensions of the suicide problem.

interesting and important implications for suicide, that is, major societal events (e.g., a war or an economic recession) which affect the suicide rate will have a *permanent* effect on the suicide rate.

It is interesting to note that we can find ideas in Durkheim's writings which are compatible with these two features of a random walk. First, Durkheim called suicide the ransom-money of civilization (Durkheim, 1951, p. 367) because the culturally-advanced European countries experienced increases in the suicide rate during the 19th Century. For example, the suicide rate rose 411 percent in Prussia from 1826 to 1890, 385 percent in France from 1826 to 1888, and 318 percent in German Austria from 1841 to 1877. The extent of the increase in the suicide rate in those days seems to suggest that the basic nature of the suicidal phenomenon changed dramatically in many regions of Europe during the period. This implies that the suicide rate may not be a stationary time series over long periods of time.

Second, social regulation and social integration were the two fundamental concepts proposed by Durkheim (1897) in his theory of the etiology of suicide. Regulation refers to a "spirit of discipline" and integration to "attachment to social groups" (Besnard, 1988). Both concepts are long-term variables because both seem to be the result of interactions among people in the community and because the formation of both discipline and social groups involves a process of trial-and-error over a long period of time.[7] It is interesting to note that, when confronted with both long and short-term perspectives, Durkheim seemed to emphasize the long-term perspective. For example, in his discussion of anomie, Durkheim was mainly interested in and preoccupied by chronic anomie rather than acute anomie (Besnard, 1988). Anomie, according to Durkheim, results from a lack of social regulation.[8]

---

[7] This does not exclude the observation that some events of a short-term nature may still increase the risk of suicide. It has been documented that the correlation between unemployment and suicide is positive when it is statistically significant (Platt, 1984; Lester and Yang, 1997; Yang, 1992). In addition, suicidologists also acknowledge that publicity of suicide stories by the media is a major cause of an immediate, short-term, increase in the suicide rate (Bollen and Phillips, 1982; Phillips, 1974, 1989; Wasserman, 1984).

[8] There seems to be a dispute among contemporary sociologists about the meaning of the concept of anomie as used by Durkheim. Merton (1957, 1964) maintained that anomie results from a disjunction between culturally prescribed goals and socially institutionalized means for achieving these goals. Besnard (1988) argued, on the other hand, that anomie is a situation

Even though detailed annual data were not available for testing the nonstationarity of the European suicide rates in the 19th Century, it would be interesting to see whether the hypothesis is supported by modern data. The existence of a unit root in the time-series suicide rate for recent American suicide rates was explored, since a nonstationary stochastic process with a unit root implies that the suicide rate follows a random walk. This, in turn, would support that hypothesis that suicide is a chronic process.

Yang (1992) suggested that a possible test procedure for this would involve two steps. First, the sample autocorrelations of the time-series suicide rate were examined. The sample autocorrelations will indicate whether the time-series follows an autoregressive stochastic process, a moving-average stochastic process, or a mix of the two, namely, an autoregressive moving-average stochastic process. The autocorrelations also indicate whether the time-series is stationary or not. Second, the Dickey-Fuller test (Dickey & Fuller, 1981) was employed to test directly whether the suicide rate has a unit root.

## TEST RESULTS

Since the sample autocorrelation functions of all of the suicide rates for the United States from 1933 to 1987 examined in Yang's study followed a gradual decay pattern instead of oscillation between consecutive lags, this provided empirical support for the autoregressive model rather than the moving-average model or the autoregressive moving-average model (Box & Jenkins, 1970; Pindyck & Rubinfeld, 1981). Secondly, the sample autocorrelation functions of all of the suicide rates examined took ten to twenty years to become zero, and this raised doubts about the stationarity of the annual time-series suicide rate. Both conclusions suggested the need for the Dickey-Fuller test. The results of the Dickey-Fuller test for the total

---

characterized by "indeterminate goals and unlimited aspirations.....in a context of expansion or increasing upward mobility." It is interesting to note that Merton's definition is more static in nature whereas Besnard's provides a dynamic dimension. Therefore, the two views can be taken as complementary aspects of the same theoretical framework.

population and for different sociodemographic groups supported the hypothesis that the time-series suicide rates are a second-order autoregressive process with a unit root (without drift).[9]

Yang also applied the same Dickey-Fuller test to the monthly suicide rates for the total population of the United States for the period 1957 to 1986 and obtained evidence for the same conclusion as for the results for the annual suicide rate. In order to explore this phenomenon further, the two-step test was applied to the annual Australian suicide rates for the total population, for males, and for females for the time period 1901 to 1985, using data obtained from Hassan and Tan (1989). The results of the tests matched exactly those for the United States data, namely, the autocorrelation functions of those three time-series decayed to zero with a lag of nine to twenty years, and the time-series appeared to fit a random walk process. Unfortunately, monthly data for Australian suicides were not available for examination.

## CONCLUSION

If the annual suicide rate is a random walk process, then any disturbance to the societal suicide rate will have a permanent impact. As a consequence, the annual suicide rate has the properties of a long-term or chronic process. This random walk hypothesis of the suicide rate is supported by Durkheim's theory of suicide, for Durkheim explicitly mentioned that social regulation tended to take time to have an impact on the societal suicide rate (Durkheim, 1951).[10]

The support for the random walk hypothesis for the annual suicide rate provided by the annual American and Australian data implies that traumatic events at the societal level will have a permanent long-term effect. It also

---

[9] Yang studied the time-series suicide rates for six age groups and four sex-by-race groups.

[7] It is not clear whether Durkheim thought that social integration could also be a chronic process. On the other hand, Durkheim mentioned that the way in which industrial revolution affected the society clearly illustrated how social regulation could change over a long period.

highlights the importance of chronic processes as a major determinant of the societal suicide rate.

The implication of these results for suicide prevention is that governments should focus on actions which will have a major impact on the society, for disturbances to the societal suicide rate will probably have a permanent impact. In England, for example, the switch from toxic coal gas for domestic use to natural gas led to a large decrease in the suicide rate, and England has continued to have a low suicide rate subsequently. Lester (1992) has shown that states in America which instituted programs to prevent youth suicide witnessed a beneficial change in youth suicide rates. These programs included legislation, Governor involvement, commission task forces, manuals and brochures, school curricula, training conferences, direct services and special studies. This study suggests the kinds of government initiatives which may have a long-term impact on suicide rates. Governments should also consider the potential impact of major changes in the social and economic conditions of the society on the suicide rate.

A recent article in *The Economist* (Anon, 2018) reported that suicide rates have declined in almost every region and every country in the world, except for the United States. This decline was attributed to the improving quality of life for Chinese and Indian women, urbanization and the decline in poverty, the imposition of controls on production and distribution of alcohol in Russia (together with price increases), limitations on the availability of lethal means for suicide (such as limiting the quantity per bottle of medications that are used for overdosing and packing the pills in plastic blisters), and less sensational reporting of suicides by the media. All of these tactics are often government policies, and they are aimed at the population of a whole rather than high risk individuals, tactics suggested by Goldney (2003) for nations with a high suicide rate (see Chapter 11) and by Lester and Yang (2006).

## REFERENCES

Anon. (2018). Defeating despair. *The Economist*, *429*, (9119, November 24), 50-53.

Besnard, P. (1988). The true nature of anomie. *Sociological Theory*, *6*(1), 91-95.

Bollen, K. & Phillips, D. P. (1982). Imitative suicides. *American Sociological Review*, *47*, 802-809.

Box, G. E. P. & Jenkins, G. M. (1970). *Time series analysis: forecasting and control*. San Francisco: Holden-Day.

Dickey, D. A. & Fuller, W. A. (1981). Likelihood ratio statistics for autoregressive time series with a unit root. *Econometrica*, *49*, 1057-72.

Diebold, F. X. & Nerlove, M. (1990). Unit roots in economic time series: a selective survey. In T. B. Fomby & G. F. Rhodes, (Eds.) *Advances in econometrics: cointegration, spurious regressions, and unit roots*, Volume *8*, pp. 3-69. Greenwich, CT: JAI press.

Durkheim, E. (1897). *Le Suicide* [*Suicide*]. Paris: Felix Alcan.

Goldney, R. D. (2003). A novel integrated knowledge explanation of factors leading to suicide. *New Ideas in Psychology*, *21*, 141-146.

Hassan, R. & Tan, G. (1989). Suicide trends in Australia, 1901-1985: analysis of sex differentials. *Suicide & Life-Threatening Behavior*, *19*, 362-380.

Kleidon, A. W. (1986). Variance bounds tests and stock price valuation models. *Journal of Political Economy*, *12*, 141-53.

Lester, D. (1989). *Suicide from a sociological perspective*. Springfield, I: Charles Thomas.

Lester, D. (1992). State initiatives in addressing youth suicide. *Social Psychiatry & Psychiatric Epidemiology*, *27*, 75-77.

Lester, D. & Yang, B. (1997). *The economy and suicide*. Hauppauge, NY, US: Nova Science Publishers.

Lester, D. & Yang, B. (2006). Should suicide prevention programs target individuals or society as a whole? *Crisis*, *27*, 200-201.

Meese, R. A. & Singleton, K. J. (1983). On unit roots and the empirical modeling of exchange rates. *International Economic Review*, *24*, 1029-35.

Merton, R. K. (1957). *Social theory and social structure*. New York: Free Press.

Merton, R. K. (1964). Anomie, anomia and social interaction. In M. B. Clinard (Ed.) *Anomia and deviant behavior*, pp. 213-243. New York: Free Press.

Motohashi, Y. (1990). Circadian variations in suicide attempts in Tokyo from 1978 to 1985. *Suicide & Life-Threatening Behavior*, *20*, 352-361.

Nelson, C. R. & Plosser, C. I. (1982). Trends and random walks in macroeconomic time series. *Journal of Monetary Economics*, *10*, 139-162.

Phillips, D. P. (1989). Recent advances in suicidology: the study of imitative suicide. In R. F. W. Diekstra, R. Maris, S. Platt, A. Schmidtke, & G. Sonneck, (Eds.) *Suicide and its prevention*, pp. 299-312. Leiden, the Netherlands: Brill.

Pindyck, R. S. & Rubinfeld, D. L. (1981). *Econometric models and economic forecasts. 2nd Edition*. New York: McGraw-Hill.

Platt, S. D. (1984). Unemployment and suicidal behavior. *Social Science & Medicine*, *19*, 93-115.

Rudebusch, G. D. (1990). Trends and random walks in macroeconomic time series: a reexamination. Paper presented at the *annual meeting of the American Economic Association*, Washington, DC.

Samuelson, P. A. (1965). Proof that properly anticipated prices fluctuate randomly. *Industrial Management Review*, *6*, 41-50.

Samuelson, P. A. (1973). Proof that properly discounted present values of assets vibrate randomly. *Bell Journal of Economics & Management Science*, *4*, 369-74.

Wasserman, I. (1984). Imitation and suicide. *American Sociological Review*, *49*, 427-436.

Yang, B. (1992). Is the time-series suicide rate of the U.S.A. a random walk? Paper presented at the *annual meeting of the American Economic Association*, New Orleans, LA.

In: The End of Suicidology
Editor: David Lester
ISBN: 978-1-53615-310-1


*Chapter 13*

# CAN MURDERERS PROVIDE CLUES TO SUICIDE?

***David Lester, PhD***
Stockton University, Galloway, New Jersey, US

Although Durkheim's (1897) theory of suicide has enormous popularity among sociologists and sociological suicidologists, I have always thought that Henry and Short's (1954) theory of suicide was more useful for two reasons (Lester, 1968). First, it combined sociological and psychological variables in predicting suicide and, second, it compared these variables as predictors of both suicide and homicide, behaviors in which aggression is directed inwardly versus outwardly, respectively. In my reviews of research and theory concerning suicide from 1897 to 1997, I found only one study that compared suicides and murderers.

Pokomy (1965) looked at self-directed and other-directed aggression when complete and when partial, by examining data about murderers, people who assaulted others (but did not kill them), completed suicides, and attempted suicides. He examined differences in place of occurrence of the act, the census tract of residence, the hour, day, and month of the act, the age of the individual, the race of the person, and the sex of the person. He found that the murderers were similar to the assaulters in all characteristics. The murderers and the completed suicides differed in all characteristics except that of sex. The completed suicides differed from the attempted suicides in hour and day of the act, age, and sex. Pokomy concluded that murder and suicide are committed by different types of people. Those who attempted suicide appeared to be a mixed group. They resembled the completed suicide group in place of occurrence of the act, their race and the census tract that they dwelt in, but they resembled the murderers in the hour and day of the act and in age. They were different from all three other groups in the high proportion of women. The problem with this study is concerns the variables studied. The variables are socio-demographic characteristics of the individuals and the timing of the aggressive act. We need studies of the psychological and psychiatric state of the four groups of individuals.

The majority of scholars focus their attention on a small segment of the scholarly universe, and so they remain relatively unaware of research and theory in neighboring segments. (Of course, the enormous scholarly output in modern times now precludes scholars from being too comprehensive in what they peruse and read outside of their particular field.) Lester (1990) examined the major theories of criminal behavior to explore whether they could be applied usefully to suicidal behavior. These theories of criminal behavior are: classic theories, positivist-individualistic theories, social structure theories (which include culture deviance theories and strain theories), learning theories (including neutralization theories), social control theories (including containment theories), social reaction theories, and social conflict theories.

## A Classical Theory of Suicide

A *classical theory* of suicide would view suicide as a rational decision made by an individual who weighs the costs and benefits of suicide versus other alternative actions. This viewpoint in suicide has rarely been proposed. However, Yang, an economist, has proposed a cost-benefit and a demand-supply analysis of suicide which is based upon such a viewpoint (Lester &

Yang, 1997). In addition, Clarke and Lester (1989) argued that the choice of a method for suicide is a rational choice based upon consideration of the effects of different methods on the body and on the mind.

## A Positivist Individualistic Theory of Suicide

*Positivist individualistic theories* of suicide would include the majority of psychological and psychiatric theories proposed to account for suicide. Such theories look for the causes of suicide in the individual's physiological constitution, psychological characteristics and psychiatric state.

## A Social Structure Theory of Suicide

Two variants of a *social structure theory* of suicide can be proposed. In a *culture deviance theory* of suicide, it would be proposed that there exist suicidal subcultures, especially in small communities such as schools, psychiatric hospitals and prisons, or Native American reservations. These subcultures have different values and attitudes from the mainstream culture. In addition, broader subcultural patterns may exist, such as the use of guns to solve problems (in both murder and suicide), which characterize whole regions (such as the southern or honor states of the United States). For example, for a long time, Hungary had the highest suicide rate of any nation in the world. In addition, Hungarian immigrants to other nations had the highest suicide rates of all immigrant groups. Perhaps Hungarians had a subculture which makes suicide more likely?

*Strain theories* of suicide would focus on the emotional experiences of those who have difficulty working toward the culturally-approved goals by socially acceptable means. Those who fail in this task will experience anger, frustration and despair. They become *retreatists*, to use Robert Merton's (1957) proposed set of types, perhaps episodically.

## A Learning Theory of Suicide

*Learning theories* of suicide have been proposed only quite recently. Lester (1987a) presented a convincing case that learning factors may play a strong role in the appearance of suicide in distressed individuals. Related to learning theories, a *neutralization theory* of suicide would focus on the ways in which the potential suicide neutralizes the inhibitions against killing himself. Interestingly, very little research has been conducted on this latter issue, and it would appear to merit more intensive study in the future. If we could find how people decrease their inhibitions against choosing suicide, we might obtain some ideas as to how these inhibitions might be increased.

## A Social Control Theory of Suicide

A *social control theory* of suicide would focus on the social bonds and internal controls which prevent people from choosing suicide. The major sociological theory of suicide, that proposed by Durkheim (1897), fits here. Durkheim proposed that social integration and social regulation, in moderation, both served to make suicide less likely. Thus, increased social bonding should make suicide less likely. Psychological theories of suicide too have recognized the importance of social bonds, such as good relationships with parents, spouse and lovers, children and friends.

One variant of the social control theories, *containment theory*, would focus in addition on the internal forces that inhibit the appearance of suicidal behavior, such as strong ego strength and a positive self-image, belief in an internal locus of control, good frustration tolerance and low impulsivity.

## A Social Reaction Theory of Suicide

A *social reaction theory* of suicide would focus on the ways in which people might be labeled as suicidal in the society and how they react to this labeling. Do they reject it or do they accept it and enter the career of being suicidal? It has been noted that putting patients on suicide alert in institutions (in order to monitor them more closely so as to prevent suicide) may result in labeling, as might happen to clients who decide to call a suicide prevention center.[1] Suicide education programs may introduce people to the suicidal career and show them how to proceed in the career.

## A Social Conflict Theory of Suicide

A social conflict theory of suicide would view suicide as the result of oppression of one group in the society by another group. Suicidal behavior may help distressed individuals who feel oppressed by others to manipulate the power balance in their relationships. Hendin (1982) has argued that the oppression resulting from racism and social class may play a role in the high rates of suicide in young urban black males.

## Discussion

Lester (1990) presented seven perspectives for viewing suicidal behavior based on the major theories of criminal behavior. Although elements of some of these perspectives have appeared in recent years, only two of the perspectives (individualistic positivist and social control) have any substantial parallels in standard suicide theorizing. Two of the perspectives were completely new. Virtually no consideration has been given by suicidologists to social reaction and social conflict perspectives. Lester did not argue that such perspectives will assume great importance in the future. Rather he suggested that consideration of the perspectives may stimulate new research into the etiology of suicidal behavior.

---

[1] At the suicide prevention center in Buffalo, where I worked from 1969-1971, we opened a *problems in living* hotline so that callers did not have to label themselves as suicidal in order to call us.

## Theories of Violence and Their Potential Relevance for Suicide

French (1991) noted that violence is often associated with substance abuse, particularly with alcohol abuse, and that there is often evidence of the involvement of neurological factors. Violence can be a symptom of a clinical syndrome, and French suggested that the generic disorder of *impulsive aggression* was most relevant to the appearance of violence in people and, in particular, the specific syndrome of *organic aggressive syndrome*, a syndrome which is thought to have an innate biochemical etiology. This syndrome was call *episodic dyscontrol* by Menninger and Mayman (1956) and was called *personality disorder- explosive type* in DSM-III. Another syndrome associated with violence, more commonly found in young people, is *post-traumatic stress disorder* linked to physical trauma (which itself might have also caused brain damage). French noted that impulsive aggression is also common in those with abnormal brain scans and, especially, epilepsy.

According to French, impulsive aggressive disorders have an early onset, and research has shown that those who have such disorders were often victims of physical and sexual abuse. These early traumata may affect the levels of neurotransmitters in the brain, including dopamine and norepinephrine, which may in turn lead to paranoid ideation and a flight-or-fight response mode in the central nervous system. These disorders are marked by unpredictability and unprovoked explosive anger. If substance abuse is present also, the drugs may act to lower the threshold for action, exacerbating both the onset and intensity of the violence. The relevant question here is whether the syndromes described by French might be applicable to suicidal behavior.

Nell (1990) described a syndrome which he called *rage dyscontrol*, that is, irritability, anger or rage in response to relatively trivial stimuli, sometimes to the extent of assault and murder, and which can be exacerbated by alcohol use. This maladaptive pattern can become chronic and characteristic of an individual's life. Nell reviewed the theories that have been proposed to account for rage dyscontrol, and he suggested the possibility of limbic system involvement. Limbic activation, often undetectable by surface electroencephalography, can cloud consciousness, diminish inhibitory control and permit the release of aggressive urges. Some rage dyscontrol individuals report altered states of consciousness during the episodes and may have partial amnesia for their actions, which supports Nell's proposal. Damage resulting from traumatic brain injury may also lead to the rage dyscontrol syndrome. Nell reviewed research on minimal brain dysfunction (or attention deficit disorder) in children that indicated that this may be common in the childhoods of those who later show rage dyscontrol in adulthood. Many individuals with rage dyscontrol have parents characterized by psychiatric disorders, alcohol abuse and violence.

## Early Physical and Sexual Abuse

In discussing possible sources of adverse childhood stressors, Knox (2008) noted that physical, emotional, and sexual abuse are risk factors for suicide (Ystgaard et al., 2004). For example, Smith and Crawford (1986) found that high school students who had attempted suicide had experienced a greater frequency of physical beatings, rapes and sexual abuse than the other students. Kaplan, et al. (1995) found that a history of attempted suicide in psychiatric outpatients was associated with sexual abuse, especially at a younger age and by a parent, with physical abuse, especially by a parent, and with physical assaults.[2]

## Epilepsy

Several reviews of the research literature have concluded that suicidal behavior is especially common in epileptics (Barraclough, 1987). Barraclough suggested that the increased risk of suicide in epileptics might

[2] The relationship between hypothalamic-pituitary-adrenal axis (HPA axis) hyperactivity and suicidal behavior may help to explain a number of risk factors for suicidal behavior such as childhood sexual abuse and traumatic life events (Gunn, 2014).

be a result of the accompanying psychiatric disturbance, substance abuse or personality disorder caused by the epilepsy.

## Substance Abuse

There is a large body of research on the association between alcohol use and abuse and suicidal behavior (Lester, 2000), both as a trait variable and as a state variable. Pernanen (1991), in a discussion of why *current* alcohol intoxication was associated with externally-directed violence reviewed three theories.

The *severity hypothesis* argues that the alcohol makes violence more extreme and more severe. Thus, more violent acts are committed, and the degree of injury should be greater. The *indiscrimination hypothesis* argues that alcohol reduces the attention of the violent individual to the social situation and norms governing it. Thus, the violence will be more inappropriate, such as taking place in public and with unacceptable victims (for example, women and children). The elicitation hypothesis argues that alcohol makes violent behavior easier to instigate, that is, intoxicated individuals will become violent in response to a lesser provoking stimulus than will the sober individuals.

These three hypotheses appear to be equally applicable to suicidal individuals who direct their aggression inwardly. French's focus on the neurological etiology of violence suggests that alcohol may increase the likelihood of violence, both internally-directed and externally-directed, because of its effects on neurological structures and processes.

## Violence in Suicidal Individuals

Although it has been tempting in the past to view suicidal individuals as not externally violent, since they appear to be directing their aggression inwardly, research does not support this view. Lester (1987b) reviewed the research on aggression in suicidal individuals. The research indicated that attempted suicides were more angry and hostile than non-suicidal psychiatric patients, and that completed suicides had shown more evidence of violence toward others and toward property compared to psychiatric patient controls.

Ellis (1987) proposed a theory of criminal behavior in which he stressed the role of testosterone in provoking violence and other criminal behavior. Lester (1993) noted that testosterone could explain the higher suicide rate in men found in almost every country in the world, which is primarily a result of a higher rate of suicide in men using violent methods for suicide. Incidentally, in the 1980s, Lester (!986) found that male suicides with tattoos were more likely to use firearms for suicide and, in that era, violent criminals were more likely to have tattoos than non-violent criminals.

## Borderline Personality Disorder

Research has documented a high incidence of suicidal behavior in those diagnosed with borderline personality disorder, a disorder also commonly associated with externally-directed violence. Research has shown that patients with a diagnosis of borderline personality disorder have a high rate of subsequent attempted suicide (Mehlum, et al., 1994) and completed suicide (Links, et al., 1990).

## Socialization

Lester (1987a) proposed a theory of suicide as the result of a failure in socialization. Suicide is a rare event, and so suicides are deviating from cultural norms. Durkheim (1897) saw suicide as more likely in those who were not integrated into or regulated by the society, calling these types of suicide egoistic and anomic, respectively. McCulloch and Philip (1967, 1972) found that attempted suicides in Scotland had shown more deviant behavior, such as juvenile delinquent behavior, and were more often living in distressed conditions (overcrowding and taken into government care).

## Discussion

The proposal in this chapter is that research into suicidal behavior should explore theories of violent behavior directed toward others for their relevance to suicidal behavior, or at least to some subgroups of suicides. Furthermore, rather than using psychiatric patients in general or healthy individuals as comparison groups in suicide research, the use of outwardly-violent comparison groups would be of great interest.

A study by Dumais, et al. (2005) supports the ideas presented in this chapter. In a psychological autopsy in Canada, they compared those suicides using violent methods with those using non-violent methods (overdoses, poisons, gas and drowning). Those suicides who used violent methods for suicide had a greater level of lifetime aggression, as well as a higher level of impulsivity. The use of violent methods was also associated with lifetime substance abuse or dependence.[3]

## References

Barraclough, B. M. (1987). The suicide rate of epilepsy. *Acta Psychiatrica Scandinavica*, *76*, 339-345.

Clarke, R. V. & Lester, D. (1989). *Suicide: closing the exits*. New York: Springer-Verlag.

Dumais, A., Lesage, A. D., Lalovic, A., Seguin, M., Tousignant, M., Chawky, N. & Turecki, G. (2005). Is violent method suicide a behavioral marker of lifetime aggression? *American Journal of Psychiatry*, *162*, 1375-1378.

Durkheim, E. (1897). *Le suicide* [*Suicide*]. Paris, France: Felix Alcan.

Ellis, L. (1987). Relationships of criminality and psychopathy with eight other apparent manifestations of sub-optimal arousal. *Personality & Individual Differences*, *8*, 905-925.

[3] The use of violent methods was also associated with psychotic disorders.

French, L. (1991). Neuropsychology of violence. *Corrective & Social Psychiatry*, *37*(1), 12-17.

Gunn, J. F. (2014). The pathophysiology of suicidal behavior. In J. F. Gunn & D. Lester, *Theories of suicide*, pp. 189-210. Springfield, IL: Charles C. Thomas,

Hendin, H. (1982). *Suicide in America*. New York: Norton.

Henry, A. F. & Short, J. F. (1954). *Suicide and homicide*. Glencoe, IL: Free Press.

Kaplan, M. L., Asnis, G. M., Lipschitz, D. C. & Chorney, F. (1995). Suicidal behavior and abuse in psychiatric outpatients. *Comprehensive Psychiatry*, *36*, 229-235.

Knox, K. L. (2008). Epidemiology of the relationship between traumatic experience and suicidal behaviors. *PTSD Research Quarterly*, *19*(4), 1-8.

Lester, D. (1968). Henry and Short on suicide: a critique. *Journal of Psychology*, *70*, 179-186.

Lester, D. (1986). Tattoos, eye color and method for suicide. *Activitas Nervosa Superior*, *28*, 239-240.

Lester, D. (1987a). *Suicide as a learned behavior*. Springfield, IL: Charles C. Thomas.

Lester, D. (1987b). Murders and suicide: Are they polar opposites? *Behavioral Sciences & the Law*, *5*, 49-60.

Lester, D. (1989). *Suicide from a sociological perspective*. Springfield, IL: Charles C. Thomas.

Lester, D. (1990). *Understanding and preventing suicide: new perspectives*. Springfield, IL: Charles C. Thomas.

Lester, D. (1992). Rage dyscontrol and suicide. *South African Journal of Psychology*, *22*, 27-28.

Lester, D. (1993). Testosterone and suicide. *Personality & Individual Differences*, *15*, 347-348.

Lester, D. (2000). *Why people kill themselves, 4th edition*. Springfield, IL: Charles C. Thomas.

Lester, D. & Yang, B. (1997). *The economy and suicide*. Hauppauge, NY, US: Nova Science Publishers.

Links, P. S., Mitton, J. E. & Steiner, M. (1990). Predicting outcome for borderline personality disorder. *Comprehensive Psychiatry*, *31*, 490-498.

McCulloch, J. W. & Philip, A. E. (1967). Social variables in attempted suicide. *Acta Psychiatrica Scandinavica*, *43*, 341-356.

McCulloch, J. W. & Philip, A. E. (1972). *Suicidal behavior*. New York: Pergamon.

Mehlum, L., Friis, S., Vaglum, P. & Kartervd, S. (1994). The longitudinal patterns of suicidal behavior in borderline personality disorder. *Acta Psychiatrica Scandinavica*, *90*, 124-130.

Menninger, K. & Mayman, M. (1956). Episodic dyscontrol. *Bulletin of the Menninger Clinic, 20*, 153-165.

Merton, R. (1957). *Social theory and social structure*. Glencoe, IL: Free Press.

Nell, V. (1990). Rage dyscontrol. *South African Journal of Psychology*, *20*, 235-242.

Pokorny, A. D. (1965). Human violence. *Journal of Criminal Law, Criminology & Police Science*, *56*, 488-497.

Smith, K. & Crawford, S. (1986). Suicidal behavior among normal high school students. *Suicide & Life-Threatening Behavior*, *16*, 313-325.

Ystgaard, M., Hestetun, I., Loeb, M. & Mehlum, L. (2004). Is there a specific relationship between childhood sexual and physical abuse and repeated suicidal behavior? *Child Abuse & Neglect*, *28*, 863-875.

In: The End of Suicidology
Editor: David Lester
ISBN: 978-1-53615-310-1


*Chapter 14*

# THE SOCIAL RELATIONSHIPS OF SUICIDAL INDIVIDUALS: A NEGLECTED ISSUE

***Dmitri I. Shustov, MD, PhD[1,*], Olga D. Tuchina[2,†] and David Lester, PhD[3,‡]***

[1]I. P. Pavlov Ryazan State Medical University, Ryazan, Russia
[2]Moscow Treatment and Research Center for Substance Abuse Disorders, Moscow, Russia
[3]Stockton University, Galloway, New Jersey, US

As was noted in Chapter 1 above, the social relationships of suicidal individuals have been a neglected issue in recent research on suicidal individuals. Lester (1972) was able to find a few doctoral dissertations that explored these relationships (e.g., Hattem, 1964), but such research is time-consuming to conduct and, in this age of publish or perish, not conducive to advancing careers. There are however, case studies that provide clues to understanding the suicidal individual. Some of these case studies were

* Corresponding Author's Email: dmitri_shustov@mail.ru
† Corresponding Author's Email: olga-shustova@yandex.ru
‡ Corresponding Author's Email: david.lester@stockton.edu

provided by Joseph Richman (1986) with his emphasis on family therapy. For example, Rosenbaum and Richman (1970) documented the hostility and death wishes of family members when talking to a family member in the hospital after attempting suicide.

Lester (1969), in a study of individuals who had attempted or threatened suicide, found that the suicidal individuals were more dependent (on an MMPI scale) than controls, and they also scored higher on a scale to measure resentment. They were asked to indicate to which of 21 significant others they would turn to for help in a variety of crisis. They were also asked on two occasions, separated by a period of time, to rate these significant others as to how much they liked them and how much they resented them. The suicidal individuals turned to significant others less often in those crises, that is, they had fewer resources. In their liking and resentment ratings, the suicidal individuals were more likely to resent those people that they had earlier rated as liking. Thus, they showed more ambivalence toward their resources than did the non-suicidal individuals.

In this chapter, we present some cases that also illuminate the role of interpersonal relationships in the appearance of suicidal behavior from the perspective of transactional analysis. We will first present two case studies.

## Two Case Studies

### Elias

Elias was 33-years-old and diagnosed with alcohol dependence (2nd stage) with heavy drinking episodes. Elias's fraternal grandfather went missing, and his uncle died from alcohol intoxication ("He drank himself to death"). At the age of 33, his alcohol-dependent father stabbed himself during a family row in front of his relatives while intoxicated. Elias was four years old and witnessed this scene. He remembered his aunt's words addressing his father, "Drop dead! You have been torturing everyone for so long."

The circumstances of Elias' birth remain unclear, but Elias thinks that he was a wanted child. The women in the family (mother and grandmother) called the newborn Elias, but his drunken father registered the boy as George (which was the father's own name). Despite the fact that the boy's formal name was George, his parents kept on calling him Elias, and Elias introduced himself as "Elias George." Following his father's death, Elias's mother, always-busy and always-absent, took care of the boy. Elias failed to recall any pleasant childhood memories. Elias idealized his father's image and claims that he has forgotten his mother whom he sees very infrequently, although they live near each other. Elias married, and took care of a stepson. (He and his wife had no children together after ten years of marriage.)

Elias reported having regular alcohol overdoses accompanied by total amnesia. He frequently got into accidents resulting in severe brain injuries (and had needed a craniotomy). Elias had once tried to burn his body with an iron, and he had tried drugs. Elias reported feelings of "shame that is hard to understand" and lonesomeness. At the age of 25, during a heavy drinking episode, one of his relatives said, "You are spoiling our life; drop dead," and he had a vision of his father's recumbent body covered with blood lying on a bed. At that point, he had the thought, "Why was my father able [to do it], and why shall I fail?", and he stubbed himself with a kitchen knife through the heart, just as his father did. He needed surgery and a long rehabilitation. At the age of 33, he applied for psychotherapy for his alcohol dependence for the first time.

Elias's self-destructive script has developed throughout his life in several domains. When he was 25, Elias replicated his father's self-stabbing. By giving Elias his own name, the father unconsciously anticipated a similarity between his own and his son's destinies. Elias' mother insisted on changing the child's name, hoping (again unconsciously) to provide Elias with a not very efficient protective (anti-suicidal) counter to his father's curse. The message was, "Don't be like your father" or "You'll stay alive as long as you aren't like your father". This message stabilized Elias' psyche until he was 25.

Elias' psychotherapy dealt with clarification of this script and the subsequent making of a no-suicide contract. Elias received one 45-minute supportive psychotherapy session every six months, and the follow-up treatment has lasted for three years with no self-destructive behavior and a stable remission of his alcohol dependence.

## Peter

Peter, 55-years- old, was diagnosed with alcohol dependence, but he succeeded in developing a twenty-year-long remission. Peter received supportive sessions from his psychotherapist every six months.

Peter's father (Alan) had two twin male siblings (born on May 15) who died from pneumonia on May 15 at the age of four months. Peter's father (also born on May 15) named his two other sons after the diseased brothers – John and Peter. Both John and Peter became alcoholics. At the age of 38 years old, the younger son, John, was faced with serious troubles. He was a casino gambler and had accumulated debts, and criminals were harassing him. Under the influence of alcohol, John strangled his girlfriend and hanged himself - on May 15. The autopsy revealed a blood alcohol concentration level of 2.7%. Peter gave the name of "Alan" to his younger son to honor his father, and his son died from pneumonia at the age of 4 months (like Alan's twin siblings) on May 15.

As a result, Peter has treated May 15 as a neurotic fetish, and made jokes to his therapist that he would "die soon on May 15". When answering a straightforward question regarding the time of his death, he said that he wanted to live until the age of 82. During the same psychotherapy session, he agreed to continue treatment for his alcohol dependence for another ten years and not to use alcohol during that period. He made a comment that "thereupon, one can die". In ten years, he will be 65. Thus, Peter has two possible death options – at 82 (which he has voiced) and at 65 (which he has concealed).

### Discussion

After a client in transactional analysis undergoes an analysis of his or her ego states (Parent, Adult and Child), and an analysis of the games that they play (Berne, 1964), they may undergo a script analysis, analyzing their life plan which is conceptualized as if it were a script for a role in a play. This life plan is developed from childhood experiences, statements made to the child (or overheard by the child) about him, stories listened to or read, and movies and television shows, viewed.

The cases above illustrates the role of scripts in the suicidal and alcoholic lives of Elias and Peter and, in particular, the role of the parents and relatives in unwittingly shaping this script. These cases also illustrate the concept of *an episcript* (English, 1969), which is a script passed on by a carrier (in the present cases, a father) to a recipient (in these cases, a son), which English called a *hot-potato game*. Episcripts are possible only when people are dependent on the episcript carrier, which was the case of Elias and Peter vis-à-vis their fathers.

## Episcripts in Families

Shustov, Merinov and Tuchina (2016) have presented cases of episcript transmission in couples. In one case, Andrew (aged 35) was diagnosed as alcohol dependent. He had been married for ten years but divorced. At the age of 21, while intoxicated, he tried to jump out of a $4^{th}$-floor window. His explanation was that he was offended by his parents, and that they would be glad if he died. He also had repeatedly cut his wrist and arms. While drunk, he provoked fights and was beaten to the point that he had been concussed. One week before his wedding, while drunk, he crashed his truck and went to the wedding ceremony with a broken arm. He promised the bride that he would stop drinking, but he broke this promise three days later.

His wife Valery (aged 36) came from a non-drinking family. She saw her main challenge as stopping Andrew drinking who, in her words, drank just a little bit. She struggled in the early years of the marriage to stop

Andrew drinking, but eventually came to view her struggle as lost. She became severely depressed and considered suicide. She swallowed a handful of various pills, but she changed her mind and vomited them up. She went into treatment and began smoking to calm herself. During the marriage, Valery had four miscarriages and surgery for an ectopic pregnancy. During the final years of her marriage, she repeatedly had suicidal thoughts.

When Valery experienced her crises, Andrew felt better, He reduced the frequency and intensity of his drinking, and he began to focus on his physical and mental health. He found a better job and had no suicidal thoughts for the next eight years of his marriage. He now saw his wife as disturbed who needed his support and help. After a divorce, Valery felt much better. She re-married and had a son. After the divorce, Andrew began drinking and having suicidal thoughts. While drunk, he tried to hang himself at work, but he was saved by his colleagues. Six months later, he was fired because of his drinking, and he moved in with his parents. He then sought treatment and was abstinent for the next three years.

Shustov, et al. (2016) saw this case as illustrating an episcript tossed back-and-forth between Andrew and Valery. When one of them was drinking and/or suicidal, the other was fine, and these phases passed from one to the other. In families with more members (especially children), more family members can participate in transmitting the episcript. Shustov et al. pointed out that episcript transmission is facilitated by inequalities between the participants so that parent-child transmission is common. Episcript transmission is also facilitated when one partner is in the role of Rescuer and the other the role of Victim. To return the episcript, they switch these roles. Finally, Shustov et al. suggested that the root of the episcript is a traumatic experience of one of the participants that remains out of awareness and wanders from one generation to another.

## DISCUSSION

There are of course many other possible interpersonal and family dynamics that may result in suicidal behavior. Episcripts are merely one type of dynamic. However, such case studies, framed within a theoretical framework (in this case Transactional Analysis), provide a much more extensive and meaningful understanding of the suicidal person than typical research in suicidology based on large samples and simplistic psychological tests and scales. This type of analysis provides a powerful argument for the importance of qualitative studies in suicidology and for research that focuses on the social and interpersonal relationships that contribute to suicidal risk and behavior.

## REFERENCES

Berne, E. (1964). *Games people play*. New York: Grove Press.

English, F. (1969). Episcript and the "hot potato" game. *Transactional Analysys Bulletin*, *8*(32), 77-82.

Hattem, J. V. (1964). Precipitating role of discordant relationships in suicidal behavior. *Dissertation Abstracts*, *25*, 1336-1336.

Lester, D. (1969). Resentment and dependency in the suicidal individual. *Journal of General Psychology*, *81*, 137-145.

Lester, D. (1972). *Why people kill themselves*. Springfield, IL: Charles Thomas.

Richman, J. (1986). *Family therapy for suicidal people*. New York: Springer.

Rosenbaum, M. & Richman, J. (1970). Suicide: The role of hostility sand death wishes from the family and significant others. *American Journal of Psychiatry*, *126*, 1652-1655.

Shustov, D. I., Merinov, A. V. & Tuichina, O. D. (2016). Episcript transmission in families of alcohol-dependent men. *Transactional Analysis Journal*, *46*(1), 13-25.

Steiner, C. (1974). *Scripts people live*. New York: Grove.

In: The End of Suicidology
Editor: David Lester

ISBN: 978-1-53615-310-1


*Chapter 15*

# The Importance of Conceptual and Theoretical Frameworks

***John F. Gunn III, PhD****

Montclair State University, Montclair, New Jersey, US

In Gunn and Lester (2014), David Lester and I argued that much research in the field of suicidology lacked theoretical grounding. However, with the popularity of some theoretical models of suicide, such as the Interpersonal-Psychological Theory of Suicide (IPTS) and the Integrated Motivational-Volitional (IMV) model, suicidology is seeing a resurgence of theoretically grounded research. These models, and many other recently proposed models of suicidal behavior, share in common the use of theoretical and conceptual frameworks to illustrate the role of concepts in the development of suicidal thoughts and behaviors. This chapter will examine the utility of conceptual and theoretical frameworks (focusing on those that are visually represented by models) in the exploration of phenomena and discuss the ways in which the field of suicidology will benefit from the continued use of such designs.

* Author's Email: john.gunn.3@gmail.com; gunnj3@montclair.edu

# Conceptual and Theoretical Frameworks

There is often some confusion concerning what is meant by a theoretical and conceptual framework, and often the two terms are used erroneously as interchangeable. This section will review what is meant by a theoretical framework and a conceptual framework, providing some detail on what distinguishes one from the other.

## Conceptual Frameworks

What is meant by the term "conceptual framework?" Conceptual frameworks have been defined a multitude of ways by a number of researchers. F. K. Lester (2005) argued that they serve the function of illustrating that the "argument that the concepts chosen for investigation, and any anticipated relationship among them, will be appropriate and useful given the research problem under investigation" (F. K. Lester, 2005, p. 460). Maxwell (1996) defined it as "the system of concepts, assumptions, expectations, beliefs, and theories that supports and informs your research…" (Maxwell, 1996, p. 25). Finally, Miles and Huberman (1984) define a conceptual framework as explaining "either graphically or in a narrative form, the main things to be studied – the key factors, constructs or variables – and the presumed relationships between them" (Miles & Huberman, 1984, p. 18).

Based on these definitions, conceptual frameworks are used to explain the relationship between concepts or constructs and their ultimate impact on the phenomena under study (e.g., suicidal thoughts and/or behaviors). Ngulube, Mathipa, and Gumbo (2015), in reviewing multiple definitions of conceptual frameworks devised a list of characteristics for conceptual frameworks:

1. Conceptual frameworks can provide motivation for concept selection and linking them to the problem under study.

2. They are sets of concepts and aspects of theory that help to establish a coherent research agenda.
3. They are less developed than theories.
4. They provide direction for research.
5. They provide a visual representation of how concepts are related to each other and the phenomena under study.
6. The link abstract concepts to empirical data.

Conceptual frameworks can be drawn directly from theoretical frameworks, although they are typically used to focus on specific aspects of those theoretical frameworks. Conceptual frameworks can serve to provide a context in which to interpret findings, as well as explain the observations found, and they can lead to the development of theory.

## Theoretical Frameworks

What is meant by the term "theoretical framework?" Theoretical frameworks have been defined as "any empirical or quasi-empirical theory of social and/or psychological processes, at a variety of levels… that can be applied to the understanding of phenomena" (Anfara, 2008, p. 871), and as "a collection of interrelated concepts, like a theory, but not necessarily so well worked-out" which "guides your research, determining what things you will measure, and what statistical relationship you will look for" (Borgatti, 1996). Theoretical frameworks are typically used to inform methodology in empirical research and provide a synthesis of the scholarly literature (Ngulube, et al., 2015).

One of the benefits of a theoretical framework is the synthesis of existing lower level theories, allowing researchers to link together theories concerning phenomena that could be related. Theoretical frameworks also allow for the stimulation of research, and they establish structured connections between observations and facts. Ngulube and colleagues (2015) highlight a number of characteristics/qualities of theoretical frameworks:

1. They serve as a basis for planning research.
2. The link research/studies to the larger literature.
3. They shape research questions and focus the study.
4. They allow researchers to narrow down projects so that they are feasible.
5. They provide a basis for planning the data collection.
6. They aid in the interpretation of findings and in drawing generalizations to other contexts.

## Representing Conceptual and Theoretical Frameworks Graphically

Both conceptual and theoretical models can be visually represented. This allows for consumers of scientific research to more clearly understand the relationships between concepts and constructs and their ultimate relationship with the phenomena under study. These visualizations can take various forms: Venn diagrams, concept maps, integrative diagrams, and so forth (Ngulube, et al., 2015). One such method to visually represent frameworks is the path diagram. Path diagrams utilize boxes and arrows to map out the relationship between variables and are typically associated with path analysis, an extension of regression analysis. Figure 1 represents a simple path diagram:

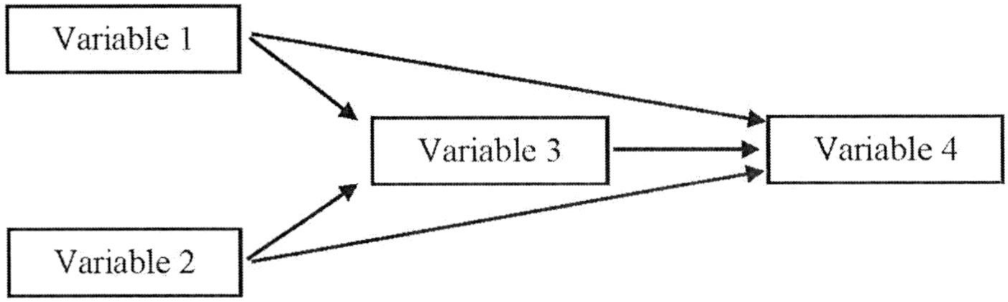


Figure 1. Example of a path diagram.

## SIMILARITIES AND DIFFERENCES

What has likely become apparent so far is that conceptual and theoretical frameworks share some similarities as well as some differences. These similarities and differences were highlighted nicely by Ngulube and colleagues (2015). They point out that both conceptual and theoretical frameworks are drawn from previous research. They both serve vital functions within research enterprises and are important for analysis within the social sciences. Some notable differences are the more abstract nature of conceptual models, which may draw from different larger theories while a theoretical model will typically focus on one overarching theory. Additionally, conceptual frameworks focus on explanation while theoretical frameworks emphasize justification (such as justification for the methodology used). Conceptual frameworks are far more common in, and better suited for, qualitative research, while theoretical frameworks are more common in, and better suited for, quantitative research (Ngulube, et al., 2015).

## FRAMEWORKS IN SUICIDOLOGY

Both forms of frameworks have been used in suicidology, although theoretical frameworks, which are typically more quantitatively applicable, have been used to a much greater extent than conceptual frameworks. Below are four contemporary theoretical frameworks being used in suicidology.

### The Interpersonal-Psychological Theory of Suicide

The Interpersonal-Psychological Theory of Suicide (IPTS) was proposed by Joiner (2005). The original theoretical framework used a Venn Diagram to illustrate the relationship between the three constructs of the model: perceived burdensomeness, thwarted belongingness, and the acquired capability for suicide. Van Orden and colleagues (2010) expanded on this model using a path diagram. In the updated model, Van Orden and colleagues introduced hopelessness and visually laid out the relationship across concepts using boxes, circles, and arrows to portray the theoretical path from the experience of thwarted belongingness, perceived burdensomeness to suicidal thoughts and behaviors.

## The Integrated Motivational-Volitional Model of Suicidal Behavior

The Integrated Motivational-Volitional (IMV) Model of Suicidal Behavior was first proposed by O'Connor (2011) and refined by O'Connor and Kirtley (2018). This model is broken into three parts (1) a pre-motivational phase, (2) a motivational phase, and (3) a volitional phase. The motivational and volitional phases are comprised of a number of boxes and arrows representing the relationships between concepts such as defeat and entrapment, suicidal ideation, and the phenomena of suicidal behavior. Additionally, there are a number of moderators represented within the model such as threats to self and motivational variables (e.g., thwarted belongingness).

## The Three-Step Model of Suicide

The Three-Step Theory (3ST) of suicide was proposed by Klonsky and May (2015) and represents a theoretical framework meant to guide research in the ideation-to-action framework put forward by Klonsky and May (2014). As the name implies, this theory postulates that three steps (represented by three question) are necessary for suicidal thoughts to transition to suicidal behavior (i.e., attempts). This model is illustrated using a box and arrow flow chart for each step with different outcomes occurring based on the answers to the three step questions. The questions for each step are:

1. Are you in pain and hopeless?
2. Is your pain greater than your connectedness?
3. Are you capable of attempting suicide?

At each of these steps, an answer of "no" or "yes" leads to different outcomes. Step one assesses ideation, with a response of "no" indicating no suicidal thoughts and an answer of "yes" indicating the occurrence of suicidal thoughts. At step 2, an answer of "no" indicates moderate suicidal thoughts, an answer of "yes" indicates stronger suicidal thoughts. Finally, at step 3 an answer of "no" indicates only the occurrence of suicidal thoughts, whereas an answer of "yes" indicates suicidal behavior occurring in the form of an attempt or death. Figure 2 represents this model visually.

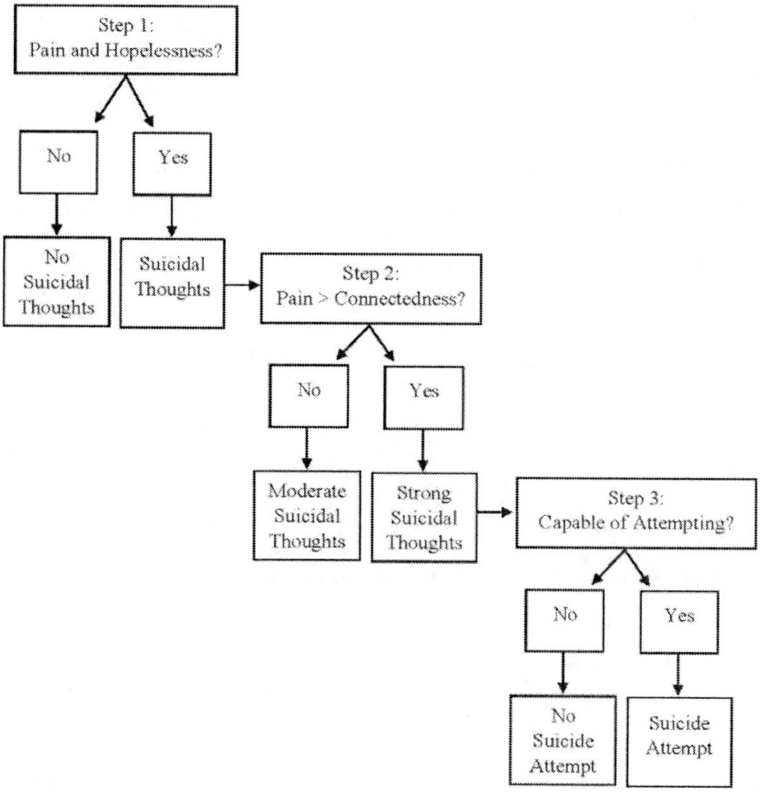


Figure 2. The 3 Step Theory. This figure is based on Klonsky & May (2015).

## The Social Pain Model of Suicide

A final model to consider is that proposed by Gunn (2017), the Social Pain Model (SPM). The SPM postulates an evolutionary origin to suicidal behavior with suicide resulting from the need to escape from the aversive experience of social and physical pain. Figure 3 is a representation of the most recent iteration of this model (Gunn, 2019). Once more a path diagram is used to outline the theorized relationship between the concepts and the target behavior, suicidal thoughts and behaviors.

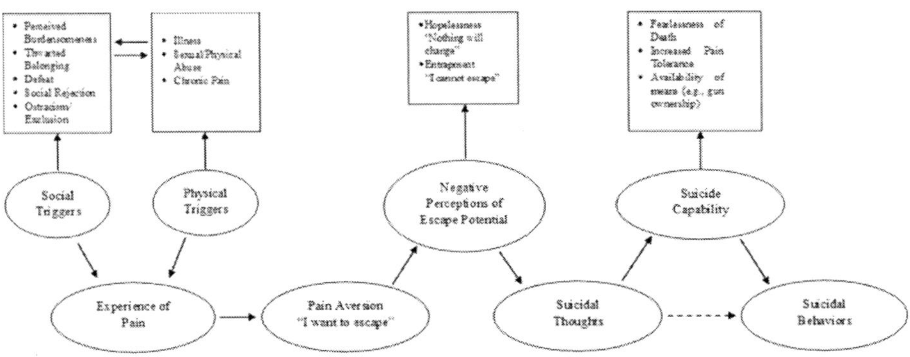


Figure 3. Social Pain Model (Gunn, 2018).

# BENEFITS OF THESE FRAMEWORKS

A number of theoretical frameworks have been outlined above that are currently in use in the field of suicidology. One question that now arises is whether or not these are of any benefit to the field. One of the immediate benefits that comes to mind in viewing these theoretical frameworks is the easily visualized and explicit assumptions that the theoretical model takes and the steps necessary for testing it. Take as an example the 3ST put forward by Klonsky and May (2015) and illustrated in Figure 2. Using this visualization, or the similar one put forward by the original authors, you can easily design a research project from which to test the theory. If the theory is to hold weight, each of the steps would need to be supported. Findings that individuals who do not experience hopelessness, for example, but who still go on to express strong suicidal thoughts or engage in suicidal behavior would challenge the assumptions put forward by the model. Each of the frameworks discussed in this chapter are laid out in such a way as to be open to validation or refutation.

Another benefit to these frameworks is that they move the field away from the mere testing of risk and protective factors through multiple regression techniques but rather lend themselves to the use of techniques that allow for causal inferences, albeit limited. Jeon (2015) discussed the use of three techniques for the examination of complex social phenomenon: multiple regression, path analysis, and structural equation modeling (SEM). In the critique of multiple regression techniques, Jeon noted that regression analyses reveal "relationships among variables, but do not imply that the relationship [is] causal" (Jeon, 2015, p. 1637). While path and SEM models also cannot speak to causality, they allow for "the tenability of the causal model formulated by a researcher" to be evaluated (Jeon, 2015, p. 1637). Path analysis and SEM also allow for the examination of direct effects, indirect effects, and total effects. Path analysis and SEM have limitations and assumptions, as do all statistical techniques, but they allow for the evaluation of theoretically grounded models when other techniques, such as multiple regression, fall short.

## References

Anfara, V. A. Jr. (2008). Theoretical frameworks. In L. M. Given (Ed.), *The SAGE Encyclopedia of Qualitative Research Methods*, pp. 869-873. Thousand Oaks, CA: Sage.

Borgatti, P. S. (1996). Elements of research. *Analytictech.* Retrieved October 12, 2019, www.analytictech.com/mb313/elements.htm.

Gunn, J. F. III. (2017). The social pain model: Understanding suicide through evolutionary psychology. *Crisis*, *38*, 281-286.

Gunn, J. F. III. (2019). *Adaptation, dysfunction, or byproduct? Placing suicide in an evolutionary context*. Manuscript in preparation.

Jeon, J. (2015). The strengths and limitations of the statistical modeling of complex social phenomenon: Focusing on SEM, path analysis, or multiple regression models. *International Journal of Social, Behavioral, Educational, Economic, Business & Industrial Engineering*, *19*, 1634-1642.

Joiner, T. E. Jr. (2005). *Why people die by suicide.* Cambridge, MA: Harvard University Press.

Klonsky, E. D. & May, A. M. (2014). Differentiating suicide attempts from suicide ideators: A critical frontier for suicidology research. *Suicide and Life-Threatening Behavior*, *44*, 1-5.

Klonsky, E. D. & May, A. M. (2015). The three-step theory (3ST): A new theory of suicide rooted in the "ideation-to-action" framework. *International Journal of Cognitive Therapy*, *8*, 114-129.

Lester, F. K. (2005). On the theoretical, conceptual, and philosophical foundations for research in mathematics education. *ZDM: Mathematics Education*, *37*, 457-467.

Maxwell, J. A. (1996). *Qualitative research design: An interactive approach.* Thousand Oaks, CA: Sage.

Miles, B. M. & Huberman, A. M. (1984). *Qualitative data analysis.* Thousand Oaks, CA: Sage.

Ngulube, P., Mathipa, E. R. & Gumbo, M. T. (2015). Theoretical and conceptual framework in the social sciences. In E. R. Mathipa & M. T. Gumbo (Eds.), *Addressing Research Challenges: Making Headway in Developing Researchers*, pp. 43-66. Noordywk, South Africa: Mosala-MASEDI Publishers & Booksellers.

O'Connor, R. C. (2011). Towards an Integrated Motivational-Volitional Model of Suicidal Behaviour. In R. C. O'Connor, S. Platt, & J. Gordon, (Eds.), *International Handbook of Suicide Prevention: Research, Policy & Practice*, pp. 181-198. Chichester: Wiley-Blackwell.

O'Connor, R. C. & Kirtley, O. J. (2018). The Integrated Motivational-Volitional Model of Suicidal Behavior. *Philosophical Transactions of the Royal Society B*, *373*.

Van Orden, K. A., Witte, T. K., Cukrowicz, K. C., Braithwaite, S. R. & Joiner, T. E. Jr. (2010). The interpersonal theory of suicide. *Psychological Review*, *117*, 575-600.

# CONCLUSION

In: The End of Suicidology
Editor: David Lester

ISBN: 978-1-53615-310-1


*Chapter 16*

# HAS SUICIDOLOGY COME TO AN END?

***David Lester, PhD***
Stockton University, Galloway, New Jersey, US

It is time to answer the question addressed by this book. Has suicidology come to an end? In one way, the answer is clearly a resounding NO. Articles, chapters and books will continue to be published in large numbers, perhaps in even increasing numbers. I did a search of PsycINFO for suicide* and found the following number of article for selected years.

| | |
|---|---|
| 1960 | 25 |
| 1970 | 118 |
| 1980 | 116 |
| 1990 | 497 |
| 2000 | 579 |
| 2010 | 1168 |
| 2017 | 1838 |

In my books *Why People Kill Themselves*, I reviewed the scholarly literature on suicide from 1897, the year of Durkheim's classic book on suicide, to 1997, using all of the search engines, from Anthropology Abstracts to PubMed. It is no wonder that I stopped at 1997. The task became too much for one person. Of course, along with this, the number of scholarly journals is increasing, with varying degrees of prestige.[1] In terms of the volume of scholarly works, the end is not in sight.

However, the important aspect of the question of whether suicidology has come to an end is whether new theories of suicide will be proposed. Some of the chapters in the present book suggest that this form of *the end* is upon us. The section on Proposed New Approaches was not encouraging. I found the critical suicidologists (Chapter 2) to be verbose but not creative, and the same goes for the attempt by Joiner and Rudd (Chapter 3) to encourage colleagues to be creative. Mostly, the contributors reviewed their own research and theories. As for Rogers and Lester (Chapter 4), their work seems to encourage the production of new research, but not necessarily new ideas.

The section on Provocative Ideas is also discouraging. Several of the chapters view suicide as inherently unpredictable and difficult, if not impossible, to understand. Bijou Yang's random walk hypothesis for the societal suicide rate (Chapter 12) casts suicide as similar to the prediction of the weather. Her model views the long-term trends in suicide rates as possibly predictable based on social changes, but the day-to-day fluctuations are random around this trend. As I write this book in the Fall, I know that next summer will be warmer, but I cannot predict the exact temperature and the daily forecast for my birthday on June 1st.

The ideas of Cas Soper (Chapter 1) are also discouraging. As I summarized one of his assertions: *there is no empirical reason to believe that predictors of suicide exist, there is no theoretical foundation for believing that risk factors exist, and there is evidence that suicide may be*

---

[1] It is my opinion that the prestige of the journal is not associated with the originality and importance of the work reported. In my reviews of scholarly research and thought on suicide, I frequently found ground-breaking work in obscure, low prestige journals and journals rarely searched by suicidologists. For example, the notion that each birth cohort may have a fixed number of suicides over its lifetime was proposed in an article in *Acta Medica et Biologica* (Uematsu, 1961).

*predictably unpredictable*. Of course, he may be wrong, but a close reading of his articles and books make a persuasive argument for his assertion.

Other provocative ideas seem only to make suicidal behavior even more of an enigma. Brian Mishara's two component mode (Chapter 5) increases the complexity of understanding suicide and, so far, has not generated any research (or interest). Chaos theory, non-linearity and tipping points (Chapter 10) also add complexity to the problem of understanding suicide and, again so far, they have not generated new research or theories.

It is noteworthy that this book has not looked at physiological research into suicidal behavior. This is, in part, a result of the fact that I view that research as a blind alley. Not only are physiological theories of psychiatric disorders quite poor but applying these theories to suicidal behavior has been even less successful. In my recent book *Rational suicide: Is it possible?* (Lester, 2014), I have argued that psychiatry as a scientific discipline has failed to produce a causal diagnostic system (and even its symptom-based system results in poor inter-psychiatrist agreement). As I have noted in my book *How Culture Shapes Suicidal Behavior* (Lester, 2019), physiologically-based theories have great difficulty understanding (or predicting) the occurrence of acts of suicide, let alone all of the other aspects of suicidal behavior, such as choice of method for suicide, motivation for the suicidal act, and all of the other factors of the suicidal act (location, timing, clothes worn, whether alcohol or drugs are ingested, etc.).

One of the results of the publish-or-perish nature of scholarly research, in which scholarly productivity is a requirement for hiring, tenure and promotion in academia, is that articles have to be published quickly and, in addition, the more prestigious universities require that these articles are published in the top scholarly journals.[2] This impedes the planning of research that might improve our knowledge of suicidal behavior. For example, long-term follow-up studies of cohorts of individuals (both at high and low risk of suicide) might throw light on the occurrence of suicide. But

[2] The top journals typically prefer substantial articles on established topics in the field. In my reviews of suicide research and my other field of interest (theories of personality), I often found that initial publication of an idea by an author in a journal such as *Psychological Reports* (in its early days of low prestige) with a follow-up article later in a journal published by the American Psychological Association.

a long-term study means that the scholarly papers will have to wait ten, twenty or more years before being written. By the time that the paper is published, the researcher will have been "non-retained."[3] In a different field, I recently communicated with those who research electroconvulsive therapy to inquire what are the long-term consequences of this practice on the brain. The longest follow-up study to date was one year!

One the most impressive long-term follow-up studies is the Terman study of gifted children which was started in 1921 by Lewis Terman at Stanford University with 1,528 gifted children, who were followed up every ten years until they all died. I was fortunate to be able to use that sample to study childhood predictors of later suicide (Lester, 1991). In the 1920s, Terman, already well-known as a developer of intelligences tests, did not have to worry about perishing.

## A Resolution

### Choice of Samples

It is hard to conduct research on those who are deceased. Psychological autopsy studies are very time-consuming and draining for the researcher. The deceased cannot be given the psychological inventories that researchers favor. But, to be honest, we are not as interested in those with suicidal ideation or those who make mild or moderate attempts at suicide as we are in those who died by suicide. Obviously, it easier to conduct research on sample of college students or samples of psychiatric patients and get data that are publishable but, if we are seriously interested in those who died by suicide, then the only meaningful individuals for research (other than suicides) are those who made lethal suicide attempts and nearly died but survived.

[3] Academics are never fired.

## Typologies

If we ever hope to better understand suicidal behavior, then we need a sound typology for suicides. To engage in research as if all suicides are alike or similar, and to look for commonalities is misguided. To assume that the suicides of individuals such as Marilyn Monroe, Herman Goring, Sigmund Freud, Yukio Mishima, George Sanders (Oscar-winning actor), and Jan Palach (who set fire to himself in 1969 to protest the invasion of Czechoslovakia by the Soviet Union) will all fit the same model is wrong. Even Sigmund Freud's suicide did not fit Freud's own theory of suicide![4]

This is illustrated by sociologists, most of whom still follow Durkheim's (1897) theory of suicide based on his typology of altruistic, egoistic, fatalistic and anomic suicide. However, I have *never* found any sociologist who used rates of those four types of suicide in his or her research. They simply use official suicide rates to test Durkheim's theory or their Durkheim-based theory which is, therefore, methodologically unsound.

Psychologists also need a typology of suicides. Researchers are often urged to compare and contrast theories. For example, does Thomas Joiner's Interpersonal Theory of Suicide (ITS) fit the data from the sample better or does the defeat-entrapment theory (DET) fit the data from the sample better? It may be instead that some suicides in the sample are ITS types while others are DET types and, in addition, there are some who do not fit into either of these pigeon holes. What types of suicides might be common?

## Predicting Suicide

Why do we need to predict suicides? And why do we do this with batteries of inventories and questions? One answer is for triage. Which clients should we focus on right now in order to prevent their suicide? In this

[4] Freud's suicide in London, England, in 1939 was motivated by the end of his long-term battle with cancer, and was not a result of anger felt toward others turned inward onto the self. Noteworthy is that his suicide was a physician-assisted suicide. Also noteworthy is that all most all textbooks on theories of personality hide this and state that Freud died of cancer (Lester, 2000).

case, a long-term, intensive psychodynamic analysis of the person would result in a more accurate prediction. However, with large number of patients, institutions (such as psychiatric clinics and hospitals) do not have enough staff to do this. Some universities screen all incoming freshmen for their mental health these days with an online survey in an effort to detect those who require a more intensive interview. Universities do not have enough counselors to give every entering freshman an intensive interview.

But we have seen in Chapter 1 that the prediction of suicidal risk is quite poor. So why do we persist? First, because poor prediction is better than no prediction. Second, because the possibility of law suits means that clinicians have to protect their practice. If a client dies by suicide and the family sues the clinician or the clinic, then it has to be shown that the clinician followed an accepted protocol. Hence the battery of inventories and questions.

Does this help us understand suicide? No.

## Understanding this Particular Suicide

I could have labeled this section *Qualitative Research*, but this tends to lead to an us-versus-them debate, with qualitative researchers feeling excluded. If we are not making greater progress in understand suicide in general, perhaps we have to be content with understanding individual suicides. It is this that led me to begin reading biographies of suicides (who had to be famous enough for someone to write a biography of them) and to write essays on them. I have read somewhere in the range of 60-80 biographies so far. They are available at http://www.drdavidlester.net/home/bibliographic-studies. I began this project because I felt that, despite my scholarly research on suicide, I had no idea why people choose to die by suicide. For some of the people whose biographies I read and wrote about (but far from all), I felt that I understood their choice and how their lives led up to that choice. Indeed, for a few, I was surprised that they lived as long as they did.

Of course, understanding one suicide may not help us understand other suicides, but understanding a few suicides might enable us to propose a typology of suicides which can then be explored empirically.

## Interpersonal Relationships

Throughout my writings, I have often stressed the absence of research on the interpersonal relationships in suicide research. Dmitri Shustov and Olga Tuchina (see Chapter 14) have provided current explorations of the interpersonal dynamics in the lives of suicides from the perspective of Transactional Analysis. We need more of this qualitative type of research, including analyses based on other systems of psychotherapy. Research on these relationships, however, is time-consuming and runs into the publish-or-perish trap.[5]

With luck, perhaps I will able to see in ten years whether suicidology ended or not.

# References

Lester, D. (1991). Completed suicide in the gifted. *Journal of Abnormal Psychology*, *100*, 604-606.

Lester, D. (2000). Freud's death from bone cancer!!!!! *Contemporary Psychology*, *45*, 233.

Lester D. (2014). *Rational suicide: Is it possible?* Hauppauge, NY: Nova Science.

Lester, D. (2019). *How Culture Shapes Suicidal Behavior*. Hauppauge, NY: Nova Science.

[5] I knew a researcher who planned to study the double-bind theory of schizophrenia by living for a month with each of a sample of families with a schizophrenic child and for a month with each of a sample of families with a normal child. His study never appeared, because he had to abandon it after a couple of families or he would never had graduated.

Uematsu, M. (1961). A statistical approach to the host factor of suicide in adolescence. *Acta Medica et Biologica, 8*, 279-286.

# Editor's Contact Information

***David Lester, PhD***
Emeritus Professor of Psychology
Stockton University, Galloway, New Jersey US
Email: david.lester@stockton.edu

# INDEX

## A



## B



## C



## D



## E

## F



## G



## H



## I



## L



## M



## N



## O



## P

## Related Nova Publications

### The Psychology of Rivalry

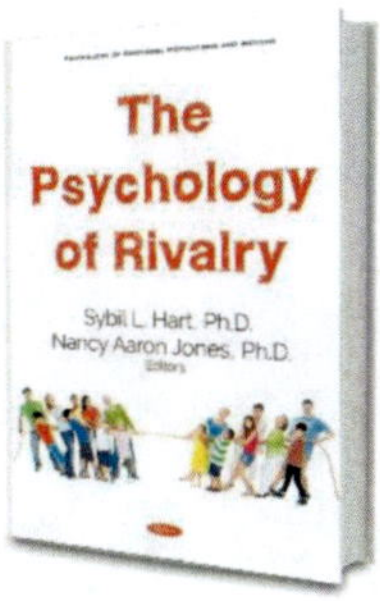


**Editors:** Sybil L. Hart, Ph.D. and Nancy Aaron Jones, Ph.D.

**Series:** Psychology of Emotions, Motivations and Actions

**Book Description:** *The Psychology of Rivalry* is an edited volume made up of chapters by leading researchers and theorists in the fields of psychology, human development, family studies, evolutionary psychology, behavioral neuroscience and genetics.

**Hardcover ISBN:** 978-1-53614-172-6
**Retail Price:** $230

### The New Science of Curiosity

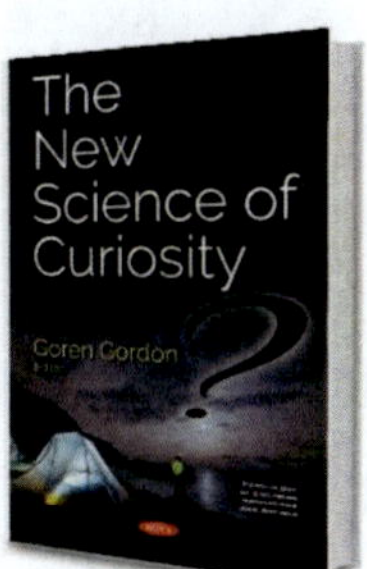


**Author:** Goren Gordon

**Series:** Psychology of Emotions, Motivations and Actions

**Book Description:** *The New Science of Curiosity* holds great promise for a better, deeper, and more comprehensive understanding of this elusive, yet crucial, aspect of human cognition. Only a multi-disciplinary diverse approach, as presented in this book, holds the key to unlocking the mysteries of exploration, seeking and investigative experiences of our grandiose dreams and daily lives.

**Hardcover ISBN:** 978-1-53613-800-9
**Retail Price:** $195

*To see complete list of Nova publications, please visit our website at www.novapublishers.com*